Library of
Davidson College

Legal Almanac Series No. 18

FAMILY PLANNING AND THE LAW

by ROY D. WEINBERG, B.A., L.L.B.
Member of the New York Bar

This legal Almanac has been revised by the Oceana Editorial Staff

Irving J. Sloan
General Editor

SECOND EDITION

**1979 Oceana Publications, Inc.
Dobbs Ferry, New York 10522**

Library of Congress Cataloging in Publication Data

Weinberg, Roy David.
  Family planning and the law.

  (Legal almanac series; no. 18)
  Published in 1968 under title: Laws governing family planning.
  Includes index.
  1. Birth control--Law and legislation--United States.
  2. Abortion--Law and legislation--United States.
  I. Title
KF3771.W4   1978   344'.73'048   78-20984
ISBN 0-379-11111-X

© Copyright 1979 by Oceana Publications, Inc.

All rights reserved. No part of this publication may be reproduced or transmitted in any form or by any means, electronic or mechanical, including photocopy, recording, xerography, or any information storage and retrieval system, without permission in writing from the publisher.

Manufactured in the United States of America.

CONTENTS

Chapter I
LEGAL ELEMENTS OF ABORTION 1

Chapter II
LEGISLATIVE AND JUDICIAL ASPECTS OF
CONTRACEPTION 29

Chapter III
LEGAL STATUS OF ARTIFICIAL
SEMINATION 69

Chapter IV
STERILIZATION AND THE LAW 77

Appendix A
AMERICAN LAW INSTITUTE, MODEL PENAL
CODE (Abortion) 91

Appendix B
SUMMARY AND ANALYSIS OF STATE LAWS
RELATING TO CONTRACEPTION 93

Appendix C
SUMMARY AND ANALYSIS OF STATE LAWS RELATING
TO VOLUNTARY STERILIZATION 98

Appendix D
SUMMARY AND ANALYSIS OF STATE LAWS RELATING
TO CONTRACEPTIVE SERVICES TO MINORS 105

ABOUT THE AUTHOR

Roy D. Weinberg is a graduate of Ohio State University and Columbia Law School. He has engaged in legal editing and research and has written on a variety of legal subjects.

Chapter I
LEGAL ELEMENTS OF ABORTION

In legal terminology, "abortion" denotes an intentional interruption of pregnancy by removal of the embryo from the womb. Properly performed by a competent obstetrician in an accredited hospital where satisfactory pre-operative and post-operative procedures are observed, it is a comparatively safe operation. However, as a result of the severe legal restriction obtaining in all American jurisdictions, most women are driven to what are at least technically illegal abortions. Although the covert character of such surgical procedures renders reliable statistical estimates difficult, there seems little doubt that criminal abortions in this country approach a figure of close to 1,000,000 annually. It has been estimated that they exceed legal abortions by a ratio of 100 to 1 and that two-thirds of those aborted are married. Technically, of course, most "legal" abortions are actually illicit in the light of the strict terms of most statutes, which authorize abortion only when necessary to preserve the life of the mother. Modern medical advances have virtually eliminated the absolute necessity of abortion to save life in the cases of most maladies formerly recognized as imperative indications for invocation of this procedure.

Ordinarily, authorized abortions are performed during the first trimester of pregnancy when it is a safe and comparatively inexpensive procedure. Such surgery is known as dilatation and curettage. The operation takes about 20 minutes and ordinarily entails hospitalization of one day. Later abortions usually involve hysterotomy, but newer procedures using concentrated oxytocin or intra-amniotic injection into the uterus of hypertonic solutions have also been employed in recent years. The latter procedures are unquestionably more hazardous than dilatation and curettage (commonly known as D & C). Even a D & C of course, is not infallible and occasional complications, including death, are inevitable. Nevertheless, the overhwelming preponderance of illegal abortions, including attempts at self-abortion and the resort to quacks, is beyond doubt the source of most fatalities. Even wealthy women, who can command the services of skilled criminal abortionists, are exposed to greater hazards than those encountered in authorized hospital abortions because of the impossiblity of ensuring adequate pre-operative and post-operative precautions under such circumstances.

LAWS GOVERNING ABORTION: At common law, abortion before "quickening" was not criminal. A few states deviated from this generally prevailing view and regarded the act as criminal at any stage of gestation. For example, in the case of Mills v. Commonwealth, 13 Pa. 630, the court held that the crime might be perpetrated from the moment "the womb is instinct with embryo life and gestation has begun" and that the rights of "an infant in ventre sa mere are fully protected at all periods after conception." The first statute making abortion a crime irrespective of "quickening" was "Lord Ellenborough's Act" (the British "Miscarriage of Women Act of 1803 (43 Geo. 3, c. 58)) which prohibited an attempt to abort by poison either before or after "quickening".

The first American law prohibiting abortion was enacted in Connecticut. This statute prohibited an attempt to abort by drugs **after** quickening and prescribed a penalty of life imprisonment as against the death penalty authorized by the British statute. In 1830, this penalty was further reduced to a term of from seven to 10 years and the purview of the law extended to include attempts to abort by means other than medication. In 1860, pre-quickening attempts were included within the scope of the prohibition, but the penalty was still further reduced to a term of from one to five years, and an attempt to abort when "necessary to preserve the life" of the mother exempted from the acts prohibited.

The original Connecticut statute was enacted in 1821.

Closely following (in 1827) was the Illinois statute, which also was restricted to the use of poisons on "any woman, being then with child," entailing a penalty, however, of not over three years imprisonment and a fine of not over $1,000. Surgical and other techniques were not mentioned in Illinois law until 1967, when the penalty also was changed to imprisonment of two to 10 years, and abortions or attempts to abort for bona fide medical or surgical purpose exempted from the law. Unlawful attempts resulting in death of the woman became murder.

The present Connecticut and Illinois laws are set forth below:

Connecticut: "Any person who gives or administers to any woman, or advises or causes her to take anything, or uses any means, with intent to procure upon her a miscarriage or abortion, unless the same is necessary to preserve her life or that of her unborn child, shall be fined not more than one thousand dollars or imprisoned in the State Prison for not more than five years or both." (Section 53-29 (Conn. Gen. Stat. Rev. (1958)

"Any woman who does or suffers anything to be done, with intent to produce upon herself miscarriage or abortion, unless necessary to preserve her life or that of her unborn child, shall be fined not more than five hundred dollars or imprisoned not more than two years or both." (Section 53-30)

Illinois: "(a) A person commits abortion when he uses any instrument, medicine, drug or other substance whatever, with the intent to procure a miscarriage of any woman. It shall not be necessary in order to commit abortion that such woman be pregnant or, if pregnant, that a miscarriage be in fact accomplished. A person convicted of abortion shall be imprisoned in the penitentiary from one to 10 years.

(b) It shall be an affirmative defense to abortion that the abortion was performed by a physician licensed to practice medicine and surgery in all its branches and in a licensed hospital or other licensed medical facility because necessary for the preservation of the woman's life." (Ill. Ann. Stat., Chapter 38, Section 23-1 (1961))

"Any person who sells or distributes any drug, medicine, instrument or other substance whatever which he knows to be an abortifacient and which is in fact an abortifacient to or for any person other than licensed physicians shall be fined not to exceed $500 or imprisoned in a penal institution other than the penitentiary not to exceed 6 months, or both." (Section 23-2)

"Any person who advertises, prints, publishes, distributes or circulates any communication through print, radio or television media advocating, advising or suggesting any act which would be a violation of any Section of this Article, shall be fined not to exceed $500 or imprisoned in a penal institution other than the penitentiary not to exceed 6 months, or both." (Section 23-3)

The original proposed draft of the 1961 Illinois amendment included three affirmative defenses which would have provided:

1. That the abortion is medically advisable because continued continuance of the pregnancy would endanger the life or gravely impair the health of the pregnant woman; or

2. That the abortion is medically advisable because the fetus would be born with a grave and irremediable physical or mental defect; or

3. The pregnancy of a woman has resulted from forcible rape or aggravated incest.

These liberal proposals, similar in substance to those of the Model Penal Code, were, however, rejected in the final draft as adopted.

The somewhat peculiar provision of the Connecticut statute regarding the preservation of the life of the "unborn child" as a qualifying exception to the general terms of the law appears also, either in identical or equivalent terms, in the statutes of a number of other jurisdictions. States having abortion statutes of this character include the following:

Minnesota	South Carolina
Missouri	Virginia
Nevada	West Virginia
New York	

The ostensible self-contradiction of legalizing abortion, which in medical terms means destroying the fetus, in cases where it is "necessary" to save or preserve the life of the "unborn child," has caused consternation in both legal and lay circles. While many attempts to explain its meaning, if any, have been made, the most logical and appealing is that it results from the failure of the law to observe the technical distinctions between abortion and premature birth or induced labor. In any case, the only coherent construction of such a provision is that it refers to premature delivery, and this conclusion is supported, for example, by a provision of the Texas statute, which provides as follows:

"If any person shall designedly administer to a pregnant woman or knowingly procure to be administered with her consent any drug or medicine, or shall use towards her any violence or means whatever externally or internally applied, and thereby procure an abortion, he shall be confined in the penitentiary not less than two nor more than five years; if it be done without her consent, the punishment shall be doubled. By abortion is meant that the life of the foetus or embryo shall be destroyed in the woman's womb or that a premature birth thereof be caused." (Article 1191, Chapter 9 (Tex. Pen. Code Ann. (1960))

Minnesota law, which includes the exception under discussion, contains comprehensive coverage of the crime of abortion. The principal pertinent provisions are the following:

"Every person who, with intent thereby to produce the miscarriage of a woman, unless the same is necessary to preserve her life, or that of the child with which she is pregnant, shall—

(1) Prescribe, supply, or administer to a woman, whether pregnant or not, or advise or cause her to take any medicine, drug, or substance; or

(2) Use, or cause to be used, any instrument or other means—shall be guilty of abortion and punished by imprisonment in the state prison for not more than four years or in a county jail for not more than one year." (Section 617.18 (Minn. Stat. Ann. (1953)

"A pregnant woman who takes any medicine, drug, or

substance, or uses or submits to the use of any instrument or other means, with intent thereby to produce her own miscarriage, unless the same is necessary to preserve her life, or that of the child whereof she is pregnant shall be punished by imprisonment in the state prison for not less than one year nor more than four years." (Section 617.19)

"Whoever shall manufacture, give, or sell an instrument, drug, or medicine, or any other substance, with intent that the same may be unlawfully used in producing the miscarriage of a woman, shall be guilty of a felony." (Section 617.20)

"Every person who shall sell, lend, or give away, or in any manner exhibit, or offer to sell, lend, or give away, or have in his possession with intent to sell, lend, give away, or advertise or offer for sale, loan, or distribution, any instrument or article, or any drug or medicine, for the prevention of conception, or for causing unlawful abortion; or shall write or print, or cause to be written or printed, a card, circular, pamphlet, advertisement, or notice of any kind, or shall give oral information, stating when, where, how, of whom, or by what means such article or medicine can be obtained or who manufactures it, shall be guilty of a gross misdemeanor, and punished by imprisonment in the county jail for not more than one year, or by a fine of not more than $500, or by both." (Section 617.25)

"Every person who shall deposit or cause to be deposited in any post-office in the state, or place in charge of any express company or other common carrier or person for transportation, any of the articles or things specified in section 617.24 or 617.25, or any circular, book, pamphlet, advertisement, or notice relating thereto, with the intent of having the same conveyed by mail, express, or in any other manner; or who shall knowingly or wilfully receive the same with intent to carry or convey it, or shall knowingly carry or convey the same by express, or in any other manner except by United States mail, shall be guilty of a misdemeanor. The provisions of this section and section 617.25 shall not be construed to apply to an article or instrument used by physicians lawfully practicing, or by their direction or prescription, for the cure or prevention of disease." (Section 26)

While the Texas law tends to confirm the suggested construction of the technically self-contradictory concept of saving a fetus by aborting it, it does so by expressly defining abortion in the same defective terms. South Carolina law, on the other hand, contains an accurate and unmistakable confirmation of this conclusion by providing that:

"Any person who shall administer to any woman with child, prescribe for any such woman or suggest to or advise or procure her to take any medicine, substance, drug or thing whatever or who shall use or employ, or advise the use or employment of, any instrument or other means of force whatever, with intent thereby to cause or procure the miscarriage, abortion or premature labor of any such woman, unless the same shall have been necessary to preserve her life or the life of such child, shall, in case the death of such child or of such woman results in whole or in part therefrom, shall be punished by imprisonment in the penitentiary for a term not more than twenty years nor less than five years. But no conviction shall be had under the provisions of this section upon the uncorroborated evidence of such woman." (Section 16-82 (S.C. Code (1952)

Section 16-84 of the same statute covers solicitation of such acts by the woman involved, but makes the crime a misdemeanor punishable by imprisonment of not over two years or fine of not over $1,000, or both, at the discretion of the court. No reference is made to the "death" of the child.

Section 16-83 is almost identical to section 16-82, except for the omission of any reference to death of the mother or child or any exception regarding the necessity of perserving the life of either. The prescribed penalty is imprisonment of not over five years or fine of not over $5,000 or both, at the discretion of the court. The reduction in degree of the offenses mentioned in 16-83 and 16-84 indicate an implicit recognition of the common law distinction between abortions before and after quickening.

In Virginia and West Virginia, the qualifying clause

respecting the saving of the life of mother or child appears separately at the close of the principal paragraph. The Virginia statute (Sections 18.1-62 and 18.1-63) (Supp. 1960) provides that:

"If any person administer to, or cause to be taken by a woman, any drug or other thing, or use means, with intent to destroy her unborn child, or to produce abortion or miscarriage, and thereby destroy such child, or produce such abortion or miscarriage, he shall be confined in the penitentiary not less than one nor more than ten years. No person, by reason of any act mentioned in this section, shall be punishable when such act is done in good faith, with the intention of saving the life of such woman or child." (Section 18.1-62)

"If any person, by publication, lecture, advertisement, or by the sale or circulation of any publication, or in any other manner, encourage or prompt the procuring of abortion or miscarriage, she shall be guilty of a misdemeanor." (Section 18.1-63)

The West Virginia law closely parallels that of Virginia, but is slightly more severe with respect to the penalty, and also provides that if the mother dies, the offender is guilty of murder. Appearing in section 5923 (W. Va. Code Ann. (1955), the Act provides:

"Any person who shall administer to, or cause to be taken by, a woman, any drug or other thing, or use any means, with intent to destroy her unborn child, or to produce such abortion or miscarriage, and shall thereby destroy such child, or produce such abortion or miscarriage, shall be guilty of a felony, and upon conviction, shall be confined in the penitentiary not less than three nor more than ten years; and if such woman die by reason of such abortion performed upon her, such person shall be guilty of murder. No person, by reason of any act mentioned in this section, shall be punishable where such act is done in good faith, with the intention of saving the life of such woman or child."

The prohibition of abortion in Nevada is set forth in several sections of the Revised Statutes of 1959. Section 200.210 provides that:

"The willful killing of any unborn quick child, by any injury committed upon the mother of such child, is manslaughter."

Submission to, or an attempt at self miscarriage, is made criminal, in the event of the death of the child, by Section 200.220 in the following terms:

"Every woman quick with child who shall take or use, or submit to the use of, any drug, medicine or substance, or any instrument or other means, with intent to procure her own miscarriage, unless the same is necessary to preserve her own life or that of the child whereof she is pregnant, and thereby causes the death of such child, shall be guilty of manslaughter."

The principal provisions respecting the crime of abortion appears in Section 201.120 as follows:

"Every person who, with intent thereby to produce the miscarriage of a woman, unless the same is necessary to preserve her life or that of the child whereof she is pregnant, shall:

1. Prescribe, supply or administer to a woman, whether pregnant or not, or advise or cause her to take any medicine, drug or substance; or

2. Use, or cause to be used, any instrument or other means, shall be guilty of abortion, and punished by imprisonment in the state prison for not more than 5 years, or in the county jail for not more than 1 year."

Nevada also (like Massachusetts, Minnesota, New York, and Washington) prohibits the manufacture of abortifacients. The pertinent provision appears in Section 201.130 as follows:

"Every person who shall manufacture, sell or give away any instrument, drug, medicine or other substance, knowing or intending that the same may be unlawfully used in procuring the miscarriage of a woman, shall be guilty of a gross misdemeanor."

The erroneous employment of the term "abortion" as a possible means of saving or preserving the life of an unborn child, the exact reverse of its true medical meaning, is by no means the only misnomer found in birth control laws. As noted in the chapter on contraceptives, the latter term is sometimes used interchangeably with prophylactics (which accurately refer only to disease prevention), and a similar confusion is occasionally found in the use of the terms "contraceptives" and "abortifacients." Abortion is possible only following conception, yet, as noted earlier, the Louisiana law apparently fails to take this into account. Its abortion statute, whose principal provisions appear in Sections 14.87 and 14.88 (La. Rev. Stat. Ann. (1950), defines and prescribes the penalties for abortion and the distribution of abortifacients.

Section 14.87 provides as follows:

"Abortion is the performance of any of the following acts, for the purpose of procuring premature delivery of the embryo or fetus:" (also involving an inaccurate definition)

"(1) Administration of any drug, potion, or any other substance to a pregnant female; or

(1) Use of any instrument or any other means whatsoever on a pregnant female.

Whoever commits the crime of abortion shall be imprisoned at hard labor for not less than one nor more than ten years."

The erroneous equating of abortifacients with contraceptives appears in the following section (14.88) which provides as follows:

"Distribution of abortifacients is the intentional:

(1) Distribution or advertisement for distribution of any drug, potion, instrument, or article for the purpose of procuring an abortion; or

(2) Publication of any advertisement or account of any secret drug or nostrum purporting to be exclusively for the use of females, for preventing conception or producing abortion or miscarriage.

Whoever commits the crime of distribution of abortifacients shall be fined not more than five hundred dollars, or imprisoned for not more than six months, or both."

The first jurisdiction to sanction a "medical" abortion was New York. Its statute of 1828 provided that:

"Every person who shall administer to any woman pregnant with a quick child, any medicine, drug or substance whatever, or shall use or employ any instrument or other means, with intent thereby to destroy such child, unless the same shall have been necessary to preserve the life of such mother, or shall have been advised by two physicians to be necessary for such purpose, shall, in case of the death of such child or of such mother be thereby produced, be deemed guilty of manslaughter in the second degree."

The present New York statutes (appearing in the Penal Law, sections 80, 81, 81-a, 82 (Article 6, "Abortion") and 1050 (Article 94, "Homicide") provide as follows:

Section 80: "A person, who, with intent thereby to procure the miscarriage of a woman, unless the same is necessary to preserve the life of the woman, or of the child with which she is pregnant, either:

1. Prescribes, supplies, or administers to a woman, whether pregnant or not, or advises or causes a woman to take any medicine, drug, or substance; or

2. Uses, or causes to be used, any instrument or other means,

Is guilty of abortion, and is punishable by imprisonment in a state prison for not more than four years, or in a county jail for not more than one year.

Section 81: "A pregnant woman, who takes any medicine, drug, or substance, or uses or submits to the use of any instrument or other means, with intent thereby to produce her own miscarriage, unless the same is necessary to preserve her life, or that of the child whereof she is pregnant, is punishable by imprisonment for not less than one year, nor more than four years."

Section 81-a: "A female who has violated section eighty-a of this article" (probably means section "eighty" as no "eighty-a" existed) "or who has committed an attempt to violate such section shall not be excused from attending and testifying or producing any evidence, documentary or otherwise, in any investigation or trial relating to violations" (of several sections relating to abortion) "or an attempt to commit any such violation, upon the ground or for the reason that the testimony or evidence, documentary or otherwise, required of her, may tend to convict her of a

11

crime or subject her to a penalty or forfeiture; but no such female shall be prosecuted or subjected to any such penalty or forfeiture for or on account of any transaction, matter or thing concerning which she is compelled, after having claimed her privilege against self-incrimination, to testify or produce evidence, documentary or otherwise, and no testimony so given or produced shall be received against her upon any criminal investigation, proceeding or trial."

Section 82: "A person who manufactures, gives or sells an instrument, a medicine or drug, or any other substance, with intent that the same may be unlawfully used in procuring the miscarriage of a woman, is guilty of a felony."

Section 1050: "Such homicide is manslaughter in the first degree, when committed without a design to effect death:

1. By a person engaged in committing, or attempting to commit a misdemeanor, affecting the person or property, either of the person killed, or of another; or

2. In the heat of passion, but in a cruel and unusual manner, or by means of a dangerous weapon."

The section then continues with the definition of first degree manslaughter in the case of abortion:

"The wilful killing of an unborn quick child, by any injury committed upon the person of the mother of such child, is manslaughter in the first degree.

A person who provides, supplies, or administers to a woman, whether pregnant or not, or who prescribes for, or advises or procures a woman to take any medicine, drug, or substance, or who uses or employs, or causes to be used or employed, any instrument or other means, with intent thereby to procure the miscarriage of a woman, unless the same is necessary to preserve her life, in case the death of the woman, or of any quick child of which she is pregnant is thereby produced, is guilty of manslaughter in the first degree."

Following New York in the recognition of "medical" abortion came Ohio, in 1834, and Missouri and Indiana, in 1835. The current statutes of these states are as follows:

Ohio: "No person shall prescribe or administer a medicine, drug, or substance, or use an instrument or other means with intent to procure the miscarriage of a woman, unless such miscarriage is necessary to preserve her life, or is advised by two physicians to be necessary for that purpose.

"Whoever violates this section, if the woman either miscarries or dies in consequence thereof, shall be imprisoned not less than one nor more than seven years." (Section 2901.16 (Ohio Rev. Code Ann.))

Missouri: "The willful killing of an unborn child, (by any injury to the mother of such child) which would be murder if it resulted in the death of such mother, shall be deemed manslaughter." (Section 559.090 (Mo. Rev. Stat. (1949))

"Any person who, with intent to produce or promote a miscarriage or abortion, advises, gives, sells or administers to a woman (whether actually pregnant or not), or who, with such intent, procures or causes her to take, any drug, medicine or article, or uses upon her, or advises to or for her the use of, any instrument or other method or device to produce a miscarriage or abortion (unless the same is necessary to preserve her life or that of an unborn child, or if such person is not a duly licensed physician, unless the said act has been advised by a duly licensed physician to be necessary for such purpose), shall, in event of the death of said woman, or any quick child, whereof she may be pregnant, being hereby occasioned, upon conviction be adjudged guilty of manslaughter, and punished accordingly; and in case no such death ensue, such person shall be guilty of the felony of abortion, and upon conviction be punished by imprisonment in the penitentiary not less than three years nor more than five years, or by imprisonment in jail not exceeding one year, or by fine not exceeding one thousand dollars, or by both such fine and imprisonment; and any practitioner of medicine or surgery, upon conviction of any such offense, as is above defined, shall be subject to have his license or authority to practice his profession as physician or surgeon in the state of Missouri revoked by the state board of medical examiners in its discretion." (Section 559.100)

Indiana: "Whoever prescribes or administers to any pregnant woman, or to any woman who he supposes to be pregnant, any drug, medicine or substance whatever, with intent thereby to procure the miscarriage of such woman, or, with like intent, uses or suggests, directs or advises the use of any instrument or means whatever, unless such miscarriage is necessary to preserve her life, shall, on conviction, if the woman miscarries, or dies in consequence thereof, be fined not less than one hundred dollars ($100) nor more than one thousand dollars ($1,000), and be imprisoned in the state prison not less than three (3) years nor more than fourteen (14) years." (Section 10-105 (Ind. Ann. Stat. (1956))

The sanctioning of abortion in the event of medical necessity—usually only where necessary to save the life of the mother, although somewhat more extensive in a few states, as will be observed—remains the single liberalizing feature of American abortion laws and has been incorporated in the statutes of most states. It is obviously inadequate, however, to meet the exigencies of countless cases of dangerous or unwanted pregnancies.

All American jurisdictions have anti-abortion statutes of varying degrees of severity. Their prohibitive provisions are all qualified, either expressly or impliedly, by certain exceptions. Four jurisdictions appear technically to be unconditional in their prohibitive terms, but closer examination discloses that exceptions exist. Louisiana, for example, specifies no circumstances under which abortion is sanctioned, but the abortion statute, considered together with the statute listing the grounds for revocation of medical licenses, may be regarded in the class of statutes sanctioning abortion where necessary to save or preserve the life of the mother. The grounds for license-revocation ennumerated include "procuring, aiding or abetting in procuring an abortion unless done for the relief of a woman whose life appears to be in peril after due consultation with another licensed physician." Massachusetts, New Jersey, and Pennsylvania also list no exceptions, but their existence appears to be implicit in the employment of the words "unlawfully" (Massachusetts and

Pennsylvania) and "without lawful justification" (New Jersey). The validity of this inference is reflected, at least in New Jersey and Massachusetts, by the holdings in State v. Brandenberg, 137 N.J.L. 124 (1948) and Commonwealth v. Brunelle, 341 Mass. 675 (1961). In the former, the court apparently recognized the right of a doctor to perform an abortion to save the life of the mother, and in the latter the right of a physician to act in the honest belief that abortion is necessary to prevent great danger to her life or health if his judgment accords with that of the "average judgment of the doctors in the community in which he practices."

Altogether, 42 jurisdictions permit abortion only when necessary to preserve the life of the mother. In 31 of these, the exception expressly appears in the statute, while in the others it is incorporated by construction. Six states sanction what may be termed "therapeutic" abortion, although their exact terminology varies. In Colorado and New Mexico abortion is permitted when necessary either to save the life of the mother or avert her serious or permanent bodily injury. Alabama, Oregon, and the District of Columbia allow abortion when necessary to preserve the mother's life or health, while Maryland provides an exception when the doctor is satisfied that "the fetus is dead, or that no other method will secure the safety of the mother."

No jurisdiction sanctions abortion for eugenic reasons (anticipated abnormality of the fetus) as indicated by rubella (German measles), radiation therapy in the early months of pregnancy, incompatibility of the Rh factor, or the use of dangerous drugs such as thalidomide by the mother, nor for sociological reasons such as pregnancy resulting from rape or incest.*

There are numerous variants among the state statutes respecting the elements constituting the crime of abortion. Although none includes the common law requirement of "quickening," this circumstance in some instances bears on the severity of the penalty. Most jurisdictions require a condition of pregnancy, either by employment of this term itself or its equivalent, such as "being with child" or "during the

---
*See Appendix for recent liberal legislation.

period of gestation." Still other statutes prohibit abortion whether the subject is "pregnant or no," or where the offender "has reason to believe" or "supposes" the woman to be pregnant.

There are also variations among the statutes with respect to recognition of the specified exceptions. Most jurisdictions require that the therapeutic necessity be factual, whereas a minority recognize the subjective element of "good faith" motivation. Even in the former, however, the defense of good faith has frequently been recognized judicially despite the literal terms of the statutes, and some states place the burden of proving non-necessity on the prosecution. Preliminary consultation with another physician or physicians is required in approximately one-third of the states.

The manufacture of abortifacients is prohibited by statute in Massachusetts, Minnesota, Nevada, New York, and Washington. Their sale is either prohibited or restricted in Colorado, Illinois, Maryland, Massachusetts, Minnesota, Mississippi, Missouri, Nevada, Rhode Island, Vermont, Washington, and the District of Columbia. Various statutes purportedly prohibit or regulate the transport, distribution, and other traffic in abortifacients, but in the light of the federal rulings respecting the Comstock Act, their validity in the case of legitimate employment is questionable.

Authority is divided as to whether a woman who submits to an abortion is an accomplice in the offense. Apparently, in the absence of statute, she is not, but some statutes specify that such complicity is criminal. Legislation of this character exists in Arizona, California, Connecticut, Idaho, Indiana, Minnesota, New York, North Dakota, Oklahoma, South Carolina, South Dakota, Utah, Washington, Wisconsin, and Wyoming. These laws, of course, pose problems in connection with prosecution of the principal offender, inasmuch as they afford a basis for refusal by the subject to testify for the prosecution on grounds of possible self-incrimination. In order to circumvent this obstacle, two states (Minnesota and Washington) have statutes providing that the privilege does not apply in such circumstances, but these laws are of dubious constitutionality. A number of other jurisdictions have dealt with the problem by granting immunity to the woman upon whom the abortion was performed. States having laws of this character include Nevada, New Jersey, New York, Ohio, and South Carolina.

Even in jurisdictions where the sole statutory exception to prohibited abortion is the necessity of preserving or saving the life of the mother, the courts frequently countenance acts which actually are designed to preserve her health, on the theory that the danger to life need not be immediate or the alternative of death certain. The necessity of such rationalizations, as well as the already noted fact that few, if any medical conditions actually require abortion to save life serves only to emphasize the confused and contradictory status of present abortion statutes, as well as the need for drastic and comprehensive reform in this area.

ABORTION LAW REFORM: Despite persistent proposals emanating from legal and medical sources for realistic reform in the area of abortion, virtually no concrete implementation of these suggestions has occurred.* In 1962 the American Law Institute approved a Model Penal Code purporting to legalize abortion in cases where:

1. Continued pregnancy would gravely impair the mother's physical or mental health.
2. The child might be born with a grave physical or mental defect.
3. Pregnancy results from rape, incest, or other felonious intercourse, including illicit intercourse with a female under the age of 16 years.

See Appendix A.

The Status of State Abortion Laws At Time of U.S. Supreme Court Landmark Decisions of *Roe v. Wade* and *Doe v. Bolton*

Although there were similarities in state abortion laws, they differed in numerous respects. These laws could be categorized as (1) the "more restrictive," (2) the "less restrictive," and (3) the "least restrictive." There is considerble variation between these arbitrary categories.

The "more restrictive" laws are those which allowed abortion only to protect the life of the pregnant woman. The thirty-one states with such laws and the dates of enactment were:

State	Enactment Date	State	Enactment Date
Arizona	1865	Nevada	1861
Connecticut	1860	New Hampshire	1848
Florida	1868	New Jersey	1849
Idaho	1863	North Dakota	1943
Illinois	1874	Ohio	1841
Indiana	1838	Oklahoma	1910
Iowa	1843	Rhode Island	1896
Kentucky	1910	South Dakota	1929
Louisiana	1914	Tennessee	1883
Maine	1840	Texas	1859
Michigan	1846	Utah	1876
Minnesota	1851	Vermont	1867
Missouri	1835	West Virginia	1848
Montana	1864	Wisconsin	1858
Nebraska	1873	Wyoming	1869

The following two states are substantially in the same grouping with some variation:

Massachusetts (1845): Court decision (1944) allowed abortion to preserve the pregnant woman's "life or health" which would otherwise be in great peril, providing the physician's belief coincides "with the average judgment of the doctors in the community in which he practices."

Pennsylvania (1860): State law prohibited "unlawful" abortions. However, "unlawful" had never been denied either by the courts or the legislature.

The "less restrictive" category of laws included those of Alabama (1951), which permitted abortion not only to preserve "life," but also "health"; Mississippi (1966), which included felonious intercourse as a justifiable reason for abortion; 11 states which had laws similar to the American Law Institute Model Abortion Law (See Appendix A); and one state, Oregon (1969), which follows the May 1968 recommendations of the American College of Obstetricians and Gynecologists.

The model Penal Code of the American Law Institute* (1962) states: "A licensed physician is justified in terminating a pregnancy if he believes that there is a substantial risk that continuance of the pregnancy would gravely impair the physical or mental health of the mother or that the child would be born with grave physical or mental defect, or that the pregnancy resulted from rape, incest or other felonious intercourse." The eleven states which have laws similar to the Law Institute model, with the dates of enactment and significant variation from the model, are:

Arkansas (1969)
California (1967) - does not have fetal indication in the law
Colorado (1967)
Delaware (1969)
Georgia (1968) - does not recognize incest as reason for an abortion
Kansas (1969)
Maryland (1968) - does not recognize incest as reason for an abortion
New Mexico (1969)

North Carolina (1967)
South Carolina (1970)
Virginia (1970)

Oregon's law, based on the recommendations of the American College of Obstetricians and Gynecologists, is essentially similar to the American Law Institute model code, but it adopted the following language: "In determining whether or not there is substantial risk....account may be taken of the mother's total environment, actual or reasonably foreseeable."

The "least restrictive" category contained those four states in which there was no legal restrictions for which an abortion may be permitted. Those four states, whose laws were all enacted in 1970, were: Alaska, Hawaii, New York and Washington. They required that the abortion must be performed by a physician and, except for New York state (it was, not incidentally, New York which was the only state in the nation which met the U.S. Supreme Court 1973 standards at the time of the landmark decisions), the abortion must be in a hospital or another approved facility.

Wisconsin, Texas, and the District of Columbia abortion laws had been declared unconstitutional by Federal District Courts even before the U.S. Supreme Court rulings.

A Woman's Right to Have an Abortion

For the past decade women and doctors have aggressively challenged the constitutionality of state abortion laws. The U.S. Supreme Court finally addressed the issue in 1973 in *Roe v. Wade* and *Doe v. Bolton*.

Jane Roe, a pregnant single woman, challenged the constitutionality of Texas criminal abortion laws which made it a crime to perform or attempt an abortion except when required to save a woman's life. She asked the court to declare the law unconstitutional and to enjoin Texas from enforcing it.

Roe claimed she (1) wanted an abortion performed by a competent licensed physician, under safe clinical conditions; (2) was unable to get an abortion in Texas because her life did not appear threatened by the continuation of her pregnancy; and (3) could not afford to travel to another state to get a legal abortion. She contended Texas law violated her rights to privacy protected by the First, Fourth, Ninth and Fourteenth Amendments to the U.S. Constitution.

The Supreme Court acknowledged the "sensitive and emotional nature of the abortion controversy" and noted that "population growth, pollution, poverty and racial overtones tend to complicate and not simplify the problem." Analyzing the history of abortion laws, the Court concluded that at the time of the adoption of our Constitution and throughout the major portion of the nineteenth century, "a woman enjoyed a substantially broader right to terminate a pregnancy than she does in most states today."

The Court found that a state criminal abortion law violates the Fourteenth Amendment when it bars abortion except to save a woman's life, without regard to the stage of pregnancy and other important interests. The right to privacy against governmental action guaranteed by the Fourteenth Amendment was "broad enough to encompass a woman's decision whether or not to terminate her pregnancy." The court, however, did not agree with the contention that a "woman's right is absolute and that she is entitled to terminate her pregnancy at whatever time, in whatever way, and for whatever reason she alone chooses." It ruled that "the abortion decision and its effectuation must be left to the medical judgment of the pregnant woman's attending physician."

The Court declined to define or base its decision on when life begins. It recognized the legitimacy of the state's interest in protecting maternal health and prenatal life but held, in accordance with constitutional principles governing the right to privacy, that a woman's right to have an abortion may only be interferred with when state interests become compelling. The Court concluded the state's interest in protecting the health of a woman did not become compelling until the end of the first trimester since during this stage an abortion is no more dangerous than childbirth. It is only beginning with the second trimester that a state may regulate abortion procedure, and then only to the extent that the regulation reasonably relates to the protection of maternal health. The Court held the state's compelling interest in protecting potential life starts at viability, usually occuring at the beginning of the third trimester, when the fetus has the "capability of meaningful life outside the mother's womb. The state may even prohibit abortions during the third trimester unless necessary to preserve the woman's health.

The *Roe* case stands for the proposition that a state criminal abortion statute that permits abortions only to save the life of a woman violates her Fourteenth Amendment right to privacy. This decision established certain constitutional standards for state abortion statutes:

(a) During the first trimester, a woman, in consultation with her physician, has the right to an abortion.

(b) During the second trimester, the state can regulate abortions as long as the regulations relate only to a woman's health.

(c) During the third trimester, regulations may also protect the potential life of the fetus, even to the point of prohibiting abortions unless necessary to preserve the woman's health.

While the Court recognized the state's power to prohibit nontherapeutic abortions in the third trimester, it nevertheless invalidated the Texas statute in its entirety, even as applied to the third trimester.

In the companion decision, *Doe v. Bolton*, Mary Doe, an indigent married Georgia citizen, together with physicians, nurses, clergy and social workers, filed suit challenging the constitutionality of certain procedural requirements of Georgia's criminal abortion laws. Doe was twenty-two years old, nine weeks pregnant, and had three children, two in a foster home and one placed for adoption becuase of Doe's poverty and inability to care for them. She had also been a mental patient at the state hospital. She was advised an abortion would be less dangerous to her health than bearing another child. Her application for a therapeutic abortion was denied. Doe claimed that this determination was a violation of her rights to privacy and liberty in matters relating to family, marriage, sex and bearing children, guaranteed at the first, Fourth, Fifth, Ninth, and Fourteenth Amendments to the U.S. Constitution.

The other plaintiffs alleged the Georgia statute "chilled and deterred" them from practicing their respective professions and deprived them of rights guaranteed by the First, Fourth, and Fourteenth Amendments.

The Georgia statute, enacted in 1968, replaced a law that had been in effect for more than ninety years. It was similar to the American Law Institute proposed abortion statute which had served as a model for legislation in several states and was considered to be a liberal, modern treatment of abortion. It prohibited abortions unless performed by a licensed Georgia physician under circumstances necessary in the physician's "best clinical judgment" to avoid danger to the woman's life or health. Plaintiffs attacked a residency requirement and three procedural conditions: (1) the abortion had to be performed in a hospital accredited by the Joint Commission on Accreditation of Hospitals; (2) the procedure had to be approved by a hospital staff abortion committee; and (3) two other physicians, by independent examination, must confirm the physician's judgment.

The Court held the three procedural conditions unduly restricted both a woman's right to privacy and a physician's practice of medicine in the following ways:

(1) The accreditation requirement was invalid because (a) Georgia had not shown only accredited hospitals could protect a woman's health during an abortion; and (b) under *Roe* there could be no regulation in the first trimester.

(2) The creation of a hospital committee on abortion, a procedure not required for other type of surgery, restricted a woman's rights which were adequately safeguarded by her own physician.

(3) The requirement of concurrence by two additional physicians (making a total of six physicians involved in the process of deciding whether a woman could have an abortion) was also unnecessarily restrictive because it had no connection with a woman's needs and infringed on a physician's practice of medicine.

Finally, the Court held the requirement, that only Georgia residents could obtain abortions in the state, also restricted a woman's constitutional right to an abortion. The state advanced no compelling interest, such as preserving state-supported facilities for Georgia residents, to justify the infringement on a woman's fundamental constitutional right to travel to another state seeking medical services.

The Court's decisions in these two cases made the laws of nearly every state either entirely or partially unconstitutional. Only New York had a law that met the Supreme Court standards in every respect even before the Court's ruling. Nine other states: Alaska, Georgia, Hawaii, Idaho, Indiana, Montana, North Carolina, Tennessee, and Washington, now have laws that place no over-all restrictions on a woman's right to have an abortion. But all are still constitutionally questionable in one or another of their procedural qualifications.

While the Supreme Court in *Doe v. Bolton* held a woman and her physician cannot be required to receive the approval of other physicians for an abortion, in *Roe v. Wade* it declined to decide whether a woman can be required to obtain spousal or parental consent. Subsequently, many states enacted legislation requiring such consent. In 1976 the Supreme Court dealt with this issue in *Planned Parenthood of Central Missouri v. Danforth*, and ruled that states may not, during the first trimester (1) require spousal consent and (2) create blanket parental consent requirements for single minors. The Court relied on the *Roe* and *Doe* cases stating that the state has no authority to veto the woman's abortion decision and therefore cannot delegate such a veto power to a spouse or parent. The Court recognized the husband's interest in his wife's pregnancy, but did not agree that providing the husband with unilateral power to veto his wife's abortion decision would serve to strengthen the marital relationship. Since the woman is more directly affected by the pregnancy, her decision to have an abortion should prevail.

Minors, like adults, possess constitutional rights, and a minor woman's privacy right, the Court stated, outweighs parents' statutory right to veto their daughter's abortion decision.

But in holding parental consent requirements unconstitutional in *Danforth*, the Court limited its ruling only to *blanket* provisions. Not every minor, the Court said, is capable of giving informed consent to an abortion. Therefore, certain abortion statutes which do not provide the minor woman with absolute unilateral decision-making authority may be constitutional.

It should be noted that while the Court did not address itself to the constitutionality of spousal and parental consent requirements for second and third trimester abortions in *Danforth*, the Court, on the same day and in light of *Danforth*, summarily affirmed a lower court judgment in *Coe v. Gerstein*, which held unconstitutional a spousal and parental consent provision not limited to any particular trimester. Several other courts, relying on the *Danforth* decision, have held unconstitutional spousal and parental requirements not confined to a particular trimester.

In 1977 the U.S. Supreme Court declared the anti-abortion statutes in Louisiana unconstitutional. A woman and her husband brought suit challenging two Louisiana criminal abortion statutes, *Raimer v. Connick*, after she had been denied an abortion in a state-supported hospital. The first statute made it a criminal offense for any person to perform any abortion for any reason, even to save the life of the pregnant woman. The second statute made it a criminal offense to advertise, distribute or sell any abortifacients.

Plaintiffs claimed the statutes were an "overboard state interference in women's right of privacy in the abortion decision." They asked the court to declare the statutes unconstitutional and to enjoin their enforcement.

The Supreme Court declared that Louisiana's statute, even more restrictive that the anti-abortion statutes it had struck down in the *Roe* and *Doe* cases in 1973, prohibiting as it did even life-saving abortions, was unconstitutional.

The statute prohibiting the advertisement, distribution and sale of abortifacients was also unconstitutional.

(It) would prohibit such acts as the original sale of medical instruments or other articles to doctors who wish to perform abortions, and their distribution by a doctor or druggist to his patient or customer. The statute contains no exceptions for abortions necessary to save the mother's life nor does it differentiate between the stages of pregnancy as does the Supreme Court's decisions in *Roe* and *Doe*.

For these reasons, this statute was unconstitutionally overboard under the authority of *Roe* and *Doe*.

Although few states have revised their abortion laws to conform with the two Supreme Court decisions (but see Appendix C for an example of a statute revised to conform "with the decisions of the United States Supreme Court. . .(and) only because of (those) decisions. . .(and) if those decisions are ever reversed or the United States Constitution is amended to allow protection of the unborn then the former policy of this State to prohibit abortions. . .shall be reinstated.), a number have acknowledged the rulings in other ways. Florida, Illinois, and Nebraska simply repealed their abortion laws and have not replaced them. Michigan and New Jersey left their laws on the books but apparently consider them void as applying to physicians performing abortions within the Supreme Court guidelines; these states would only prosecute laymen who perform abortions. Rhode Island considers its abortion law void, but has taken no further action, and Maryland has determined that its abortion laws no longer carry criminal penalties. Texas, whose law was the subject of *Roe v. Wade*, removed its law from the criminal statutes and placed it, unchanged, in the civil statutes. Hence, abortion is no longer a criminal act in Texas, although the legislature apparently does not approve of the Supreme Court's decision.

The fact is that the laws of practically every state are unconstitutional and therefore unenforceable. This means that if a woman in any of these states can find a doctor willing to perform an abortion and she and the doctor are later subject to criminal prosecution because of it, they have a defense based on the unconstitutionality of the laws under which they are being prosecuted.

abortion, or for any indecent or immoral use; or any written or printed card, letter, circular, book, pamphlet, advertisement, or notice of any kind giving information, directly or indirectly, where, how, of whom, or by what means any of such mentioned articles, matters, or things may be obtained or made; or

Whoever knowingly takes from such express company or other common carrier any matter or thing the carriage of which is herein made unlawful—

Shall be fined not more than $5,000 or imprisoned not more than five years, or both, for the first such offense and shall be fined not more than $10,000 or imprisoned not more than ten years, or both, for each such offense thereafter."

Prohibition of the importation of "immoral articles," including contraceptives, reappears in 19 U.S.C. 1305, together with the procedure prescribed for its enforcement. The text of this section, insofar as material to our study, is as follows:

"All persons are prohibited from importing into the United States from any foreign country * * * any drug or medicine or any article whatever for the prevention of conception or for causing unlawful abortion * * * ."

"Provided, That the drugs hereinbefore mentioned, when imported in bulk and not put up for any of the purposes hereinbefore specified, are excepted from the operation of this subdivision * * * "

Upon the appearance of any such * * * matter at any customs office, the same shall be seized and held by the collector to await the judgment of the district court as hereinafter provided; and no protest shall be taken to the United States Customs Court from the decision of the collector. Upon the seizure of such * * * matter the collector shall transmit information thereof to the district attorney of the district in which is situated the office at which such seizure has taken place, who shall institute proceedings in the district court for the forfeiture, confiscation, and destruction of the * * * matter seized. Upon adjudication that such * * * matter thus seized is of the character the entry of which is by this section prohibited, it shall be ordered destroyed and shall be destroyed. Upon adjudication that such * * * matter thus seized is not of the character the entry of which is by this section prohibited, it shall not be excluded from entry under the provisions of this section.

In any such proceeding any party in interest may upon demand have the facts at issue determined by a jury and any party may have an appeal or the right of review as in the case of ordinary actions or suits."

JUDICIAL CONSTRUCTION OF THE COMSTOCK ACT: The literal terms and apparent restrictive effect of the Comstock Act have, for most practical purposes, been abrogated by judicial construction in a series of landmark cases. In 1915, the medical profession was held to be exempt from the unqualified anti-abortion provisions of the Act in the case of Bours v. United States, 229 F 960 (7th Cir). In 1930, it was held in the case of Youngs Rubber Corp. v. C.I. Lee & Co., 45 F2d 103 (2nd Cir) that violation of the Comstock Act did not preclude an action under the Trademark Act, which barred actions only when trademarks were used in an unlawful business. In making this determination, the court declared:

"Taken literally, this language would seem to forbid the transportation by mail or common carrier of anything 'adapted' in the sense of being suitable or fitted, for preventing conception * * * even though the article might also be capable of legitimate uses and the sender in good faith supposed that it should be used only legitimately. Such a construction would prevent mailing to or by a physician or any drug or mechanical device adapted for contraceptive or abortifacient uses, although the physician desired to use or prescribe it for proven medical purposes. The intention to prevent a proper medical use of drugs or other articles merely because they are capable of illegal uses is not lightly to be ascribed to Congress." Observing that the Act also forbade the mailing of obscene literature, the court noted that it had never been thought to bar from the mails medical writings sent to or by physicians for legitimate purposes.

The existence of an unlawful intent as a prerequisite to conviction under the Act was proclaimed in the case of Davis v. United States, 62 F2d 473 (6th Cir (1933)). In this action, in which the defendant was a wholesale druggist, the court said:

"If we are right in our view that * * * intent that the articles * * * shipped in interstate commerece were to be used for condemned purposes is a prerequisite to conviction, it follows that there was error in refusing to admit evidence offered by the appellants tending to show good faith and absence of unlawful intent."

Whatever the impact of these earlier decisions, the case which, in effect, dealt a death blow to the Comstock Act was that of United States v. One Package, 86 F2d 737 (2nd Cir (1936)). This landmark decision declared that the contraceptive provisions of the Tariff Act of 1930—similar to those of the Comstock Act—did not apply to physicians. The court concluded that the Comstock Act was not intended "to prevent the importation, sale or carriage by mail of things which might intelligently be employed by conscientious and competent physicians for the purpose of saving life or promoting the well-being of their patients."

Several subsequent holdings have fortified and extended this viewpoint. In United States v. Nicholas, 97 F2d 510 (2nd Cir (1938)), the mailing of matter describing contraceptives was held to be legal, but the addressee had the burden of proceeding with proof that he was entitled to receive it. Contraceptive books and pamphlets, said the court, are "lawful in the hands of those who would not abuse the information they contained. This excuses the magazines addressed as they were to their local editor; being lawful in the hands of physicians, scientists and the like, the claimant at bar was their most appropriate distributor."

In Consumer's Union v. Walker, 145 F2d 33 (D.C. Cir (1944)), the mailing of a report evaluating certain contraceptive material to members of the Consumer's Union, who had submitted statements that they were married and used prophylactic materials on the advice of physicians, was declared legal on the ground that the information therein "vitally concerned the lives and health of those to whom it was directed" and that "Congress did not intend to exclude from the mails properly prepared information intended for properly qualified people."

In 1960, a federal court held that an attempt to mail vending machines and prophylactics was not violative of the Comstock Act (United States v. H.L. Blake Co., 189 F. Supp. 930 (D.C. Ark.). The court said that notations on the prophylactic packages specifying that they were sold only for prevention of disease indicated that there was no intent to supply them for the prevention of conception. The burden was on the government, as a prerequisite to conviction, to prove that the articles were mailed with a "specific intent" of being used for contraceptive purposes.

These cases make it clear that federal laws pertaining to contraceptive materials and information do not restrict their dissemination for lawful purposes related to the preservation of health and life. The sole surviving requirement of federal law would appear to be that such matter be made available only to married couples. The mere **advocacy** of contraception, of course, is protected by the Constitutional guarantee of free speech and press and should in no case be confused with the issue of dissemination of materials and information.

State Law

The enactment of the Comstock Act was followed by a series of so-called "obscenity" statutes on the state level. Legislation of this character was enacted in every state except New Mexico. Many of these laws mentioned contraceptives expressly but all were susceptible to a construction prohibiting their dissemination. Prior to the One Package decision, state as well as federal policy respecting contraception remained inflexible. Subsequent developments, however, have altered the situation radically on the state level as well.

State statutes vary widely. A number prohibit only advertising; some deal solely with the distribution of prophylactics; others restrict the dissemination of contraceptives to medical and pharmaceutical sources.

As noted at the outset, the only severely restrictive state statutes, those of Connecticut and Massachusetts, have been abrogated recently by judicial decision and repeal. Before reviewing the individual state statutes now in effect, let us examine the texts of the Connecticut and Massachusetts laws and the developments leading to their abrogation.

The Connecticut statutes invalidated in the Griswold holding provided as follows:

"Any person who uses any drug, medicinal article or instrument for the purpose of preventing conception shall be fined not less than fifty dollars or imprisoned not less than sixty days nor more than one year or be both fined and imprisoned." (Connecticut General Statutes (1958 Revised), Title 53, Ch. 939, Sec. 53-32)

"Any person who assists, abets, counsels, causes, hires, or commands another to commit any offense may be prosecuted and punished as if he were the principal offender." (Connecticut General Statutes (1958 Revised), Title 54, Ch. 959, Sec. 54-196)

Prior to the Griswold holding, many attempts to have these statutes repealed or declared unconstitutional were unsuccessful. In the case of State v. Nelson, 126 Conn. 412 (1940), the Connecticut Supreme Court of Errors sustained the conviction of two physicians and a nurse as accessories to the criminal use of contraceptive devices. In the case of Tileston v. Ullman, 129 Conn. 84 (1942), the court held that these statutes prohibit physicians from prescribing contraceptives even to save a patient's life or protect his health or welfare. An appeal to the United States Supreme Court was dismissed on technical grounds (318 U.S. 44 (1943)). In Buxton et al v. Ullman, 147 Conn. 48 (1959), which, like Tileston v. Ullman, was a declaratory judgment proceeding, the Connecticut court again upheld the constitutionality of these statutes. An appeal to the United States Supreme Court (Poe et al v. Ullman, 367 U.S. 497 (1961)) was dismissed on the ground that the statute was a "dead letter" law and not enforced. Justices Douglas and Harlan, however, dissented on the ground that the statutes constituted an unconstitutional invasion of the right of privacy incident to the intimate marital relationship. Two other Justices dissented on other grounds.

In Griswold v. Connecticut, the defendants were the executive director and medical director of the Planned Parenthood League of Connecticut, which had opened a clinic in New Haven where contraceptive information was disseminated to married persons. The defendants were charged under both statutes and convicted under the accessory Act as persons who assisted and counseled others in the use of contraceptives. After affirmance by the Connecticut Supreme Court of Errors, an appeal was taken to the United States Supreme Court, which at long last held both statutes unconstitutional on the grounds that by prohibiting the use, rather than merely regulating the sale of contraceptives they involved invasions of the right of privacy. This right, though not expressly mentioned in the Constitution, emanates, said the Court, "from the totality of the constitutional scheme under which we live." This right attaches to the intimate relations of married couples and is "adversely affected unless" considered "in a suit involving those who have this kind of confidential relation to them."

The Griswold case was decided by a seven-to-two vote, and both the concurring and dissenting opinions reflect the wide diversity of views on this controversial subject. The concurring opinion of Mr. Justice Harlan placed reliance directly on the Fourteenth Amendment, independent of any rights incorporated by reference from the Bill of Rights or the general purview of various amendments to the Constitution. Another concurring opinion, by Mr. Justice Goldberg, joined by Chief Justice Warren and Mr. Justice Brennan, relied largely on the Ninth Amendment which provides that "The enumeration in the Constitution, of certain rights, shall not be construed to deny or disparage others retained by the people." Mr. Justice White, also concurring, concluded that the purpose of the statutes—prevention of extra-marital relations—was achievable by other available and less drastic means. The two dissenting opinions—by Mr. Justice Black and Mr. Justice Stewart—stressed state's rights, separation of governmental powers, the impropriety of judicial interference with legislation based on personal views respecting its wisdom, and the absence in the Bill of Rights or elsewhere in the Constitution of any general right of privacy.

The repealed Massachusetts statute appeared in Massachusetts Annotated Laws (1956) Title 1, Ch. 272, Secs. 20 and 21. It did not prohibit the use of contraceptives, but their manufacture, sale and distribution. The texts of these sections read as follows:

Section 20

"Whoever knowingly advertises, prints, publishes, distributes or circulates, or knowingly causes to be advertised, printed, published, distributed or circulated, any pamphlet, printed paper, book, newspaper, notice, advertisement or reference, containing words of language giving or conveying any notice, hint or reference to any person, real or fictitious, from whom, or to any place, house, shop or office where any poison, drug, mixture, preparation, medicine or noxious thing, or any instrument or means whatever, or any advice, direction, information or knowledge, may be obtained for the purpose of causing or procuring a miscarriage of a woman pregnant with child or of preventing, or which is represented as intended to prevent, pregnancy, shall be punished by imprisonment in the state prison for not more than three years or in jail for not more than three years or in jail for not more than two and one half years or by a fine of not more than one thousand dollars."

Section 21

"Whoever sells, lends, gives away, exhibits, or offers to sell, lend or give away any instrument or other article intended to be used for self-abuse, or any drug, medicine, instrument or article whatever for the prevention of conception or for causing unlawful abortion, or advertises the same, or writes, prints or causes to be written or printed a card, circular, book, pamphlet, advertisement or notice of any kind stating when, where, how, of whom or by what means any such article can be purchased or obtained, or manufactures or makes any such article, shall be punished by imprisonment in the state prison for not more than five years or in jail or the house of correction for not more than two and one-half years or by a fine of not less than one hundred nor more than one thousand dollars."

The repeal of these laws in 1966 was accompanied by positive legislation authorizing physicians and pharmacists to furnish contraceptive devices and drugs, and permitting public health agencies, registered nurses, and hospital maternity clinics to give information to married persons respecting the procurement of professional advice regarding such drugs and devices. The new law includes Sections 20 and 21 in their original language, but prefaced with the words "Except as provided in Section 21A." Section 21A provides that:

"A registered physician may administer to, or prescribe for, any married person drugs or articles intended for the prevention of pregnancy or conception. A registered pharmacist actually engaged in the business of pharmacy may furnish such drugs or articles to any married person presenting a prescription from a registered physician.

A public health agency, a registered nurse, or a maternity health clinic operated by or in an accredited hospital may furnish information to any married person as to where professional advice regarding such drugs or articles may be lawfully obtained.

This section shall not be construed as affecting the provisions of sections 20 and 21 relative to prohibition of advertising of drugs or articles intended for the prevention of pregnancy or conception; nor shall this section be construed so as to permit the sale or dispensing of such drugs or articles by means of any vending machine or similar device."

While this statute represents a significant advance from the measure repealed, it is still more restrictive than the laws of other states (except Wisconsin) in confining the prescription of such drugs and articles to married persons.

RECENT REFORMS: The period attending the invalidation of the Connecticut statutes and repeal of the Massachusetts law inaugurated a new era in state legislation. In 1965, progressive measures were passed in 11 jourisdictions: California, Colorado, Florida, Illinois, Iowa, Kansas, Michigan, Minnesota, Nevada, New York, and Ohio.

California amended its "Business and Professional Code" by removing restrictions on the advertising of contraceptives and contraceptive services for public health education purposes by persons not commercially interested in the sale of contraceptives. The amended statute provides:

"Every person who wilfully writes, composes or publishes any notice or advertisement of any medicine, or means for producing or facilitating a miscarriage or abortion, or for the prevention of conception, or who offers his services by any notice, advertisement, or otherwise, to assist in the accomplishment of any such purpose is guilty of a felony and shall be punished as provided in the Penal Code. It shall not, however, be unlawful for information about the prevention of conception to be disseminated for purposes of public health education by any person who is not commercially interested, directly or indirectly, in the sale of any medicine or means which may be used for the prevention of conception." (Business and Professional Code, Section 601)

Colorado enacted a statute authorizing health and welfare departments and other governmental agencies to provide and pay for family planning services to all parents. This act, appearing in Article 20, Chapter 36, Colorado Revised Statutes 1963, provides as follows:

Family Planning and Birth Control

"36-20-1. Services to be offered by the county. The governing body of each county and each city and county or any health department thereof or any welfare department thereof may provide and pay for, and each county and each city and county or any health department thereof may offer family planning and birth control services to every parent who is a public assistance recipient and to any other parent or married person who might have interest in and benefit from such services; provided that no county or city and county or department thereof is required by this section to seek out such persons.

36-20-2. Extent of services. Such family planning and birth control services shall include interview with trained personnel; distribution of literature; referral to a licensed physician for consultation, examination, tests, medical treatment and prescription; and, to the extent so prescribed, the distribution of rhythm charts, drugs, contraceptive devices and similar products.

36-20-3. Counties may charge for services. The governmental unit making provision for and offering such service' may charge those persons to whom family planning and birth control services are rendered a fee sufficient to reimburse the county or city and county all or any portion of the costs of the services rendered.

36-20-4. Services may be refused. The refusal of any person to accept family planning and birth control services shall in no way affect the right of such person to receive public health assistance or to avail himself of any other public benefit and every person to whom such services are offered shall be so advised initially both orally and in writing. County and city and county employees engaged in this administration of this article shall recognize that the right to make decisions concerning family planning and birth control is a fundamental personal right of the individual and nothing in this article shall in any way abridge such individual right, nor shall any individual be required to state his reason for refusing the offer of family planning and birth control services.

36-20-5. In all cases where the recipient does not speak or read the English language, the services shall not be given unless the interviews shall be conducted in, and all literature shall be written in, a language which the recipient understands.

36-20-6. County employee exemption. Any county employee or city and county employee may refuse to accept the duty of offering family planning and birth control services to the extent that such duty is contrary to his personal religious beliefs, and such refusal shall not be grounds for any disciplinary action, for dismissal, for any inter-departmental transfer, for any other discrimination in his employment, or for suspension from employment with the county or city and county, or for any loss in pay or other benefits.

36-20-7. Article to be liberally construed. This article shall be liberally construed to protect the rights of all individuals to pursue their religious beliefs, to follow the dictates of their own consciences, to prevent the imposition upon any individual of practices offensive to the individual's moral standards, to respect the right of every individual to self determination in the procreation of children, and to insure a complete freedom of choice in pursuance of his constitutional rights."

In Illinois, a policy recommended earlier in the year by the Birth Control Commission of that state was implemented by legislation permitting referral for birth control information of all mothers, whether married or unmarried, including those not living with their husbands, providing they are recipients of public assistance and over the age of 15. The statute also authorizes welfare workers to **discuss** family planning with relief clients.

An amendment to the Iowa State Welfare Department appropriation bill included authorization for family planning services and reimbursement therefor. This amendment is almost identical in both form and substance to the previously mentioned Colorado statute, with the single significant distinction that it applies only to welfare recipients, whereas the Colorado measures includes **all** parents and married persons.

In Kansas, positive legislation was enacted authorizing the State Board of Public Health to establish family planning centers in cooperation with state and county welfare boards. This statute provides as follows:

"AN ACT relating to the public health and welfare; directing the state board of health to establish and maintain family planning centers to furnish and disseminate information concerning, and means and methods of planned parenthood; and prscribing the duties of the state board of social welfare and county boards of social welfare and county health departments in connection thereto.

Be it enacted by the legislature of the State of Kansas: Section 1. The state board of health may establish and maintain family planning centers in cooperation with county welfare offices and county health departments. Such family planning centers, upon request of any person who is over 18 years of age and who is married or who has been referred to said center by a licensed physician and who resides in this state, may furnish and disseminate information concerning, and means and methods of planned parenthood, including such contraceptive devices as recommended by the state board of health. Such methods and means may be consistent with the religious and personal convictions of the individual to whom furnished. Sec. 2. The state board of social welfare and the several county boards of social welfare and county health departments may cooperate with and assist the state board of health in the establishment and operation of the family planning centers required to be established and maintained by section 1 of this act. * * *."

Michigan is another state which enacted legislation implementing a policy adopted earlier in the year by a state agency—the Michigan State Welfare Commission. The following provisions were added to the Welfare and Health Laws:

Welfare Law

"Sec. 14B. The Commission, and under its supervision, county, city and district departments of social welfare, are authorized to make available upon the request of recipients of public assistance advice and treatment in family planning. Written or oral notice may be provided to such recipients of public assistance of the availability of family planning services and such notice shall include a statement that receipt of public assistance is in no way dependent upon a request or nonrequest for family planning services, provided that no effort shall be made to suggest or persuade recipients to request or not request family planning services. Such services shall be made available in accordance with rules and regulations promulgated by the commission under law, which shall include provisions for referral upon request of the recipient to a public agency or, on a contractual basis, to a private agency of the recipient's choice."

Health Law

"Sec. 7A. The State Health Commissioner, and under his supervision, health departments or boards of counties, districts and cities, may provide family planning services to medically indigent women. Written or oral notice may be provided to such medically indigent women of the availability of family planning services and such notice shall include a statement that receipt of public health services is in no way dependent upon a request or nonrequest for family planning services, provided that no effort shall be made to suggest or persuade any medically indigent woman to request or not to request family planning services. Family planning services shall be provided in accordance with rules and regulations promulgated by the Commissioner under law."

Minnesota modified its statute on "Indecent Articles and Information" by deleting the phrase "for the prevention of conception" and adding a section providing that:

"Instruments, articles, drugs, or medicines for the prevention of conception or disease may be sold, offered for sale, distributed, or dispensed only by persons or organizations recognized as dealing primarily with health or welfare. Anyone convicted of violation of this section shall be guilty of a gross misdemeanor and punished by imprisonment not to exceed one year or by a fine of not more than $500 or both."

A significant revision of the New York statute respecting contraception was also adopted in 1965. The old law, at least literally, forbade the dissemination of contraceptive information by anyone other than a physician. The section pertaining to physicians—which is retained under the new law—permits them to prescribe and dispense contraceptives and drugs, and is construed to allow trained assistants to aid the physician in such dispensation under his direction and control. The new law also removes restrictions on the dissemination of contraceptives information generally, but retains the ban on "articles * * * for causing unlawful abortion." An abortion reform bill has just been killed in committee in the present session of the legislature. The terms of this proposal are discussed in a later chapter. The 1965 revision also includes a new paragraph in the section pertaining to contraception. Penal Law, Section 1142 was amended to include the following provision:

"The sale or distribution of any instrument or article, at any recipe, drug or medicine for the prevention of conception, is authorized only by a duly licensed pharmacy, and such sale or distribution to a minor under the age of 16 years is prohibited. An advertisement or display of said articles, within or without the premises of such pharmacy, is hereby prohibited."

The most sweeping revision of all came in Ohio where all reference to the prevention of conception was removed from the criminal code, thus eliminating all restrictions on the advertisement, sale and distribution of contraceptive drugs, devices, and information. Sections 32-34 of the Ohio Revised Code were amended so as to permit unconditional advertisement and sale by anyone, whereas the pre-existing provisions entrusted such dissemination solely to responsible professional people.

The Florida welfare law was likewise amended in 1965 to clarify previously ambiguous provisions which deterred many relief recipients from requesting birth control information from fear that this might subject them to the "suitable home" law, permitting welfare authorities to take children from homes deemed "unsuitable." The reform provides that "a request for the services of a voluntary birth control program shall not be deemed" violative of the "suitable home" statute. Still, additional amendment seems advisable, in view of the fact that birth control is linked to the general punitive provisions of the "suitable home" law, which may continue to generate the same apprehensions.

In Nevada, a 1965 amendment to the state public health law directs the Division of Public Health to establish a birth control program. The sum of $23,000 was appropriated for this purpose.

The liberal legislative trend extended into 1966. Massachusetts, as already noted, repealed its highly restrictive statute and enacted legislation allowing physicians to prescribe, pharmacists to sell, and clinics to supply information respecting contraceptives. Alaska adopted a law directing its Health and Welfare Department to compile and distribute family planning information to hospitals, clinics, and individuals upon request. Georgia authorized health departments to furnish family planning services. West Virginia authorized such departments to establish family planning clinics, and Michigan passed a law authorizing social welfare departments to make certain contraceptive appliances and drugs available to relief recipients upon request, through agencies, licensed medical and osteopathic physicians, and pharmacies.

On the federal level, Congress enacted the "Food for Freedom" bill, including provisions permitting the use of surplus funds overseas for the assistance of family planning programs.

REGULATORY LEGISLATION: As indicated in the foregoing survey, the restrictive effect of both state and federal statutes has been largely neutralized by judicial abrogation, repeal, amendment, or administrative policy. There remain, nevertheless, numerous statutes—to say nothing of hundreds of local ordinances—regulating the sale, distribution, and advertisement of contraceptive or prophylactic materials, as well as the dissemination of information. Such statutes vary widely, both in scope and severity. Some restrict the distribution of contraceptives to medical and/or pharmaceutical sources. Some prohibit or regulate only advertising. Some exempt certain professional classes from their purview, and still others deal only with the distribution of prophylactics. It is important to bear in mind, however, that the literal terms of legislation of this character are not invariably accurate indications of the practical status of the law. This is frequently reflected by liberal judicial construction and administrative deviation from the law's technical requirements, as, for example, in states which include birth control services in their public health programs, notwithstanding ostensibly unqualified statutory prohibitions. Conversely, even states having no specific statutes respecting contraception nevertheless regulate such activity in varying degrees in connection with statutes bearing on comparable activities.

The state of Alabama has no statute addressed specifically to the subject of contraception or the dissemination of contraceptive information. In Thomas v. Thomas, 219 Ala. 196 (1919), it was held that a husband's conduct in preventing conception against the will of his wife and her expressed desire to have children did not constitute "cruelty" justifying divorce.

Although Tennessee likewise has no state statute repecting contraceptives or relevant information, it was held in the case of McConnell v. Knoxville, 172 Tenn. 190 (1937), that the City of Knoxville had the power to regulate by ordinance the sale of contraceptives within the city limits. However, the ordinance involved expressly exempted doctors and druggists from its coverage.

Laws Regulating Sale

A number of jurisdictions prohibit the general sale of contraceptives, but exempt physicians and/or pharmacists from the purview of the law. Among these are Arkansas, Delaware, Idaho, Montana, Oregon, and Wisconsin.

The pertinent Arkansas statute provides as follows:

"No appliances, drugs or medicinal preparations intended or having special utility for the prevention of conception or veneral diseases shall be advertised (except in periodicals, the circulation of which is substantially limited to physicians and the drug trade), displayed, sold or otherwise disposed of in the State of Arkansas, without a license therefor issued by the State Board of Pharmacy, as hereinafter provided, except that this section shall not apply to physicians and medical practitioners regularly licensed to practice medicine or osteopathy in the state of Arkansas licensed by the State Board of Medical Examiners." (Ark. Stat. (1947) Title 82, Ch. 9, Section 82-944).

A subsequent section (82-950) provides:

"It shall be unlawful for any person, firm, corporation, co-partnership or association to display or expose for sale any of the articles described in section 1" (quoted above) "of this act, or any containers or packages containing or advertising the same. It shall be unlawful to publicly advertise the sale or uses of the same on any placards, billboards, hand bills, newspapers, periodicals, signs, or other printed matter or by radio; but the prohibition of this section respecting advertising shall not apply to medical and drug publications, the circulation of which is confined substantially to physicians and the drug trade, or to literature enclosed in or around the original package."

Delaware law also exempts physicians, as well as both retail and wholesale druggists, in the following language:

"No person, except as provided in Section 2503 of this title, shall sell, give away, or otherwise distribute to the public, in stores, on the streets, by vending machine, by peddling from house to house, or in any public place or office building, or in any manner whatsoever, any appliance, drug or medicinal preparation intended or having special utility for the prevention of conception or veneral disease * * * . No person shall exhibit, display or expose for sale any appliance, drug or medicinal preparation intended or having special utility for the prevention of conception or venereal disease, or exhibit, display or expose any container, or package therefor descriptive or suggestive of the contents, or advertise the sale of the same by any placards, billboards, handbills, newspapers, periodicals, signs, or by any means of publication either visual or auditory, and either individually or by broadcast * * * ." (Del. Code Ann. (1953, Title 16, Ch. 25, Sections 2501 and 2502)

The exceptions set forth in Section 2503 are as follows:

"The prohibition expressed in Section 2501 of this title shall not apply to wholesale druggists specifically licensed by this State, to the extent that such druggists are permitted to sell or distribute appliances, drugs and medicinal preparations of the character specified in such section only to regularly licensed drug stores, and only such appliances, drugs and medicinal preparations of the character specified in such section as conspiciously bear the identification of the manufacturer thereon or on the retail container thereof; nor shall the prohibition specified in such section apply to the sale or distribution of such appliances, drugs or medicinal preparations by regularly licensed physicians in the normal and usual course of the practice of their profession; nor shall the prohibition specified in such section apply to the sale or distribution of such appliances, drugs or medicinal preparations at retail by drug stores or pharmacies, provided such sales are made from prescription counters of such drug stores or pharmacies and by a registered pharmacist there employed, and only to persons 18 years of age and upwards."

Several sections of the Idaho statutes pertain to the problem of contraception, and likewise include exceptions in the cases of physicians and pharmacists. The pertinent provisions are as follows:

"Every person who wilfully publishes any notice or advertisement of any medicine or means for producing or facilitating a miscarriage or abortion, or for the prevention of conception, or who offers his services by any notice, advertisement, or otherwise to assist in the accomplishment of any such purpose, is guilty of a felonly." (Idaho Code Annotated (1948), Title 18, Ch. 6, Sec. 18.603)

"No appliances, drugs or medicinal preparations intended or having special utility for the prevention of conception and/or venereal diseases, shall be advertised (except as hereinafter provided) displayed, dispensed, sold or otherwise disposed of in the State of Idaho, without a license issued therefor by the State Board of Pharmacy of the state of Idaho, as hereinafter provided, authorizing the sale thereof, **except that Sections 39-801—39-810 shall not apply to physi-**

cians and medical practitioners licensed to practice medicine or osteopathy or chiropractic in the state of Idaho." (Title 39, Ch. 8, Sec. 39-801) This section is implemented by the immediately following sections. Section 39-803 prohibits the conspicuous display of licenses, while 39-804 restricts the issuance of licenses to wholesale druggists, wholesale drug sundries jobbers, surgical supply houses and manufacturers of such appliance, drugs and medicinal preparations (sales are permissible only to physicians and licensees). Section 39-805 confines the issuance of retail licenses to drug stores with registered pharmacists, and the dispensation of such materials to registered pharmacists over the prescription counter (sales by machine or by house or street solicitation are prohibited). Advertising and display are prohibited by Section 39-807, with a proviso exempting medical and drug publications whose circulation is substantially confined to physicians and the drug trade, and literature enclosed in and around the original package. Pursuant to Section 38-809, suppositories, cones, tablets and simple cleansing powders not classified as contraceptives or prophylactics by the Department of Public Health or State Board of Pharmacy must be labeled "for medicinal purposes only." If thus labeled, advertising is permitted, but literature enclosed must not name or refer to any other products which are contraceptives or prophylactics, or insiduously convey to readers contraceptive or prophylactic features of other products, or convey the impression that such suppositories, cones, tablets or cleansing powder have contraceptive virtues. Any advertising "that claims the product is simply an antiseptic or cleansing agent is permissible, but such words as 'fear', 'worry', 'wives', 'married women', 'marriage hygiene', 'safe', or words of similar import, are not permissible."

The Montana law includes three sections containing provisions pertinent to the regulation of contraceptives. These are Sections 94-3609, 94-3616, and 94-3617 of Title 94, Chapter 36 (Montana Revised Codes Annotated (1947)). Section 94-3609 provides:

"Every person who wilfully writes, composes or publishes any notice or advertisement of any medicine or means of producing or facilitating a miscarriage or abortion, or for the prevention of conception, or who offers his services by any notice, advertisement or otherwise, to assist in the accomplishment of such purposes is quilty of a misdemeanor.'' The following sections, 94-3616 and 94-3617, contain restrictions on sale and advertising, with specified exceptions. Section 94-3616: "It shall be unlawful for any person, firm, corporation, co-partnership, or association to sell, offer for sale, or give away, through the medium of vending machines, personal or collected distribution, by solicitation, peddling or in any other manner whatsoever, contraceptives, devices, prophylactic rubber goods, articles for prevention of venereal diseases, and other infections, or any sex-inciting devices or contrivance in the state of Montana. **The foregoing provisions shall not apply to regularly licensed practitioners of medicine, osteopathy or other licensed persons practicing other healing arts, and registered pharmacists of the state of Montana, nor to wholesale drug jobbers or manufacturers who sell to the retail stores only."**

Section 94-3617: "It shall be unlawful to exhibit or display prophyslactics or contraceptives in any show window, upon the streets, or in any public place other than in a place of business of a licensed pharmacist, or to advertise such in any magazine, newspaper or other form of publication originating in, or published within the state of Montana; to publish or distribute from house to house or upon the streets, any circular, booklet or other form of advertising, or by other visual means, or by auditory method or by radio broadcast; or by use of outside signs in stores, billboards, window displays or other advertising visible to persons upon the streets or public highways; **provided, however, that nothing in this Act shall prevent the advertising of prophylactics or contraceptives in the trade press of those magazines whose principal circulation is to the medical and pharmaceutical professions; or to those magazines and other publications having inter-state circulation outside of the state of Montana where the advertising does not violate any United States law or Federal postal regulation; nor to the furnishing within the store or place of business of a** licensed pharmacist, to persons qualified to purchase, and then only upon their inquiry, such printed or other information as is requisite to proper use in relation to any merchandise coming within the provisions of this Act."

The Oregon law, which is quite detailed, covers advertising and sale, as well as specific requirements respecting identification, necessary information, and compliance with standards prescribed by the State Board of Pharmacy and State Board of Health. Section 435.010 (Ore. Rev. Stat (1955), Title 36, Chapter 435), relating to advertising and dispensation of contraceptives provides that:

"(1)No appliances, drugs or medicinal preparations intended or having special utility for the prevention of conception or venereal diseases or both, shall be advertised, displayed, sold or otherwise disposed of in this state without a license issued by the State Board of Pharmacy, as provided in this chapter, which licenses shall be in addition to other licenses required by law.

(2)The prohibitions of subsection (1) of this section do not apply to:

(a) **Physicians and medical practitioners regularly licensed to practice medicine or osteopathy in this state by the State Board of Medical Examiners.**

(b) **Advertisements in periodicals, the circulation of which is substantially limited to physicians and the drug trade.**

Oregon also has specific licensing requirements and those relating to identification, standards of quality, and other information respecting contraceptives. Under Section 435-090, goods of the class specified in 435.010 may be sold at retail or wholesale only if they (1) Specifically identify the manufacturer and distributor by firm name and address on the appliance and on the container in which the goods are sold or intended to be sold; (2) Comply with standards of grade and quality of such goods as are prescribed by the State Board of Pharmacy and approved by the State Board of Health. As to prophylactics, including diaphragms, rubbers and skins, each such prophylactic manufactures for sale in Oregon must bear the name and address of the manufacturer and distributor, the date of manufacture and the brand name. Under Section 435.110, no person may display or expose for sale any article mentioned in 435.010 or any containers or packages containing or advertising the same or publicly advertise the sale or uses of such articles on any placards, billboards, handbills, newspapers, periodicals, signs or other printed matter or by radio—with a proviso, however, exempting medical and drug publications whose circulation is substantially confined to physicians and the drug trade, and literature enclosed in or around the original package.

The advertisement and sale of "indecent articles" is selectively prohibited by the laws of Wisconsin. Section 151.15 of Title 15, Ch. 151 (Wis. Stat (1955) provides as follows:

"(1) As used in this chapter, the term 'indecent articles' means any drug, medicine, mixture, preparation, instrument, article or device of whatsoever nature used or intended or represented to be used to procure a miscarriage or prevent pregnancy.

(2) No person, firm or corporation shall publish, distribute or circulate any circular, card, advertisement or notice of any kind offering or advertising any indecent article for sale, nor shall exhibit or display any indecent article to the public.

(3) No person, firm or corporation shall manufacture, purchase, or rent, or have in his or its possession or under his or its control, any slot machine, or other mechanism or means so designed and constructed as to contain and hold indecent articles and to release the same upon the deposit therein of a coin or other thing of value.

(4) No person, firm or corporation shall sell or dispose of or attempt to offer to sell or dispose of any indecent articles to or for **any unmarried person;** and no sale in any case of any indecent articles shall be made **except by a pharmacist registered under the provisions of ch. 151 or a physician or surgeon duly licensed under the laws of this state.**

(5) Any person, firm or corporation violating any provision of this section shall be deemed guilty of a misdemeanor and upon conviction thereof shall be punished by a fine of not less than $100 nor more than $500 or by imprisonment in the county jail for not to exceed 6 months or by both

such fine and imprisonment."

Laws Regulating Advertising

While many state laws include provisions prohibiting or regulating the advertisement of birth control devices, those of Arizona and Pennsylvania are addressed exclusively to this area.

Section 13-213, Title 13, Chapter 2, Article 2 (Ariz. Rev. Stat. Ann. (1956) provides that:

"A person who wilfully writes, composes or publishes a notice or advertisement of any medicine or means for producing or facilitating a miscarriage or abortion, or for the prevention of conception, or who offers his services by a notice, advertisement or otherwise, to assist in the accomplishment of any such purposes, is guilty of a misdemeanor."

It was held, however, in State v. Senner, 92 Ariz. 231 (1962), that this section prohibits only the advertising of "specific trade branded devices" and not referrals by physicians or nurses to Planned Parenthood clinics or the recommendation of contraceptive devices on a "person to person" basis. Nevertheless, Arizona law appears to permit Planned Parenthood clinics to distribute literature only upon solicitation.

The pertinent Pennsylvania statute (Title 18, Ch. 2, Art. V, Sec. 4525 (Pa. Stat. Ann. (Purdon 1945)) provides that:

"Whoever prints or publishes, or causes to be printed or published, in any newspaper, pamphlet, book or circular, any advertisement of, or sells or keeps for sale, or gives away or publishes an account or description of, or by writing, publishes or circulates any notice of any secret drug, nostrum, medicine, recipe or instrument, purporting to be for the use of females for the purpose of preventing conception, or procuring abortion or miscarriage, is guilty of a misdemeanor, and shall upon conviction thereof, be sentenced to pay a fine not exceeding five hundred dollars ($500), or undergo imprisonment not exceeding one (1) year, or both.

Nothing contained in this section shall be construed to apply to teaching in regularly chartered medical colleges, or the publication of standard medical books."

A number of cases make it clear that this statute prohibits only the publication or exhibition of contraceptive articles. In <u>Commonwealth v. Mosholder,</u> 46 D & C 31, 91 P.L.J. 139 (Cambria County 1943), it was held that the keeping of a quantity of diaphrams in a car trunk and garage did not constitute a violation of the law, since the sale or keeping for sale of contraceptives is not now prohibited so long as the articles are neither publicized or exhibited. In <u>Commonwealth v. Rupp,</u> 47 D & C 302, 91 P.L.J. 100 (Alleghany County 1943), the statute was held not to prohibit the sale of condoms. The court also said that such sales did not constitute a common law offense injurious to public morals. In <u>Commonwealth v. Payne,</u> 66 D & C 462 (Beaver County 1948), it was held that the law did not prohibit the sale (or keeping for sale) of contraceptives, so long as they were in no way publicized or exhibited.

Missouri law provides for the seizure of contraceptive devices and informative material, but also contains a section dealing in detail with advertising. Section 563-300, Title 38, Chapter 563 (Mo. Rev. Stat. (1949) provides as follows:

"If any person shall print or publish, or cause to be printed or published, in any newspaper in this state, any advertisement of any secret drug or nostrum purporting to be for the use of females, or if any druggist or other person shall sell or keep for sale or shall give away any such secret drug or nostrum purporting to be for the use of females, or if any person shall by printing or writing, or in any other way, publish an account or description of any drug, medicine, instrument or apparatus for the purpose of preventing conception, procuring abortion or miscarriage, or shall by writing or printing, or any circulars, newspaper, pamphlet or book, or in other way, publish or circulate any obscene notice or shall, within this state, keep for sale or gratuitous distribution, any secret drug, nostrum or medicine for the purpose of preventing conception, procuring abortion or miscarriage, such person or persons so violating any of the provisions of sections 563.280 and 563.290 shall be deemed guilty of a misdemeanor, and shall, upon conviction thereof, be fined in any sum not exceeding one thousand dollars, or be imprisoned in the county jail not exceeding six months, or both, at the discretion of the court; **provided, nothing herein shall be construed to affect teaching in regularly chartered medical colleges, or the publication of standard medical books."**

Sale by Vending Machine

The last quoted statute has an almost identical counterpart in the laws of Nebraska, except that the first sentence of the provision begins "If the publishers of any newspapers shall print or publish any advertisement", etc. Nebraska law, however, also prohibits the sale or other disposition of **prophylactics** by vending machine, or in any case except under duly authorized license (except in the case of physicians selling or disposing to patients in the regular practice of their profession, and not in the manner specified for a licensee) (Neb. Rev. Stat. (Reissue 1956) Chapter 71, Article 11, Section 71-1106). It is also unlawful in Nebraska to show or display prophylactics in any show window, on the streets or in any public place, but a licensee may show or display such merchandise within his place of business (Section 71-1113).

Hawaii, Maryland, New Jersey (by judicial construction), North Dakota, South Dakota, Utah, and Virginia likewise prohibit the sale of contraceptives and/or prophylactics by vending machine.

Section 302A, Title 31 (Hawaii Rev. Laws (1955) prohibits the public sale of prophylactics by mechanical coin-operated vending machines. (Hawaiian law also restricts advertising in comprehensive terms found in Section 155-73, Title 21 (Hawaii Rev. Laws (1955) as follows: "No person shall display any outdoor advertising giving or purporting to give information from whom or where medicines may be obtained for the cure, prevention or treatment of diseases peculiar to females, venereal diseases or impotence, sterility, gonorrhea, gleet, stricture, syphilis, abortion or miscarriage, or articles or means of preventing conception, or containing pictures or illustrations of an immoral character.")

Maryland law prohibits the sale of contraceptives by vending machine, with the somewhat puzzling exception of "places where alcoholic beverages are sold for consumption on the premises." This statute provides that it is:

"unlawful for any person, firm or corporation to sell or offer for sale any contraceptive device by means of a vending machine or other automatic device whether or not such contraceptive is advertised as such or as a prophylactic, except in places where alcoholic beverages are sold for consumption on the premises. This exception not to include railroad stations, air and bus terminals. Nor shall it include places where alcoholic beverages are sold for consumption on the premises in Howard County.". Violation of this law is punishable by a fine of not over $1,000 for each offense. The use of each such vending machine or other automatic device is declared to constitute a separate offense.

North Dakota law specifically prohibits the sale of contraceptives by vending machines as follows:

"The offering for sale, distribution or other disposition by means of a vending machine or other automatic machine of drugs, medicines, or devices for the prevention of disease or pregnancy is expressly prohibited. Possession of such machines by a person, firm or corporation in his place of business shall be prima facie evidence of sale. Any such machines shall be destroyed on order of a magistrate when found in violation hereof, and the possessor shall be guilty of a misdemeanor and shall be punished by imprisonment in the county jail for not more than thirty days or by a fine or not more than one hundred dollars or by both such fine fine and imprisonment." (Section 12-43-12, Title 12, Chapter 12-43 (N.D. Stat.)

South Dakota likewise forbids the sale of contraceptives. The statute provides as follows:

"No person, firm or corporation shall publish, distribute or circulate any circular, card, advertisement or notice of any kind offering or advertising any prophylactic for sale, nor shall exhibit or display any prophylactic to the public.

No person, firm or corporation shall manufacture, purchase or rent, or have in his possession or under his or its control, any vending machine, or other mechanism or means so designed or constructed as to contain and hold any prophylactic and to release the same upon the deposit therein of a coin or other thing of value.

As used in this section the word 'prophylactic' means any article or device of whatsoever nature intended or having special utility for preventing pregnancy or venereal disease.

Any person, firm or corporation violating any provision of this chapter shall be deemed guilty of a misdemeanor and upon conviction thereof shall be punished by a fine not to exceed one hundred dollars or thirty days in the county jail, or by both such fine and imprisonment. In addition thereto, any license, permit or registration certificate issued under any law or ordinance to any such persons, firm or corporation shall be cancelled or revoked." (Section 13.1726, Title 13, Chapter 13.17 (S.D. Code (1952)

(Louisiana law, Section 14-18, Title 14, Chapter 1 (La. Rev. Stat. Ann (1950) provides that the "Distribution of Abortifacients is the intentional: (1) Distribution or advertisement for distribution of any drug, potion, instrument, or article for the purpose of procuring an abortion; or (2) Publication of any advertisement or account of any secret drug or nostrum purporting to be exclusively for the use of females, for preventing conception or producing abortion or miscarriage." (punishable by fine of not over $500 or imprisonment for not over six months, or both).

Utah law prohibits the use of vending machines, but is addressed solely to the sale, display, advertising, etc. of **prophylactics.** This statute (Section 58-19-2, Title 58, Chapter 19 (Utah Code Ann. (1953) provides that:

"It shall be unlawful to be in possession of to sell, give away, or otherwise dispose of prophylactics except by a licensee under the conditions specified in sections 58-19-7 and 58-19-8, and the use of any mechanical device or vending machine in connection with such sales or disposition, is prohibited; **provided, however, that physicians are ex-**

empted from the provisions of this act when disposition or sale is made in the regular practice of their profession and to their patients, and when such sale or disposition is not made in the manner specified for a licensee."

The prescribed standards of quality for authorized articles for sale are set forth in Section 58-19-5 as follows:

"Only such goods of the class specified in section 58-19-2 shall be sold in this state so as to specifically identify the manufacturer thereof on the appliance or on the container in which the goods are sold or are intended to be sold, whether at wholesale or retail, nor shall any such goods be sold in this state unless the same shall comply with the standards as to such goods, respecting grade and quality, which may be approved by the state board of health. The board shall adopt the following standards * * * ."

The requirements respecting display and advertising are set forth in Section 58-19-10 as follows:

"It shall be unlawful to show or display prophylactics in any show window facing a public street, highway or passageway, upon the streets or in any public place, or to advertise in any magazine, newspaper or other form of publication, originating in, or published within the state of Utah, to distribute from house to house or upon the streets, any circular, booklet or other form of advertising, or by visual means or auditory method or by radio broadcast; or by the use of outside signs on stores, billboards, window display or other advertising visible to persons upon the street or public highway.

Provided, however, that nothing in this act shall prevent the advertising of prophylactics in the trade press or those magazines whose principal circulation is to the medical and pharmaceutical professions; to those magazines and other publications having interestate circulation, originating outside of the state of Utah where the advertising does not violate any United States law or federal postal regulation; nor to the furnishing within the store or place of business of a licensee, to persons qualified to purchase such printed or other information as is needed in relation to any prophylactics coming within the provisions of this act."

Virginia legislation is similar to that of Utah with respect to subject matter, i.e., regulations relating to the sale of prophylactics, but the specific provisions are somewhat different. Section 18.1-203 of Title 18, Chapter 4 (Va. Code Ann. (1950) contains the following provisions:

"(1) No drug, medicinal preparation, appliance, device or other article intended or having special utility for the prevention of venereal disease, hereinafter referred to as device, shall be sold or otherwise disposed of in this State except by duly licensed practitioners of medicine; and in pharmacies and retail outlets. Pharmacies and retail stores desiring to sell such devices shall apply in writing to the State Board of Pharmacy and the Board shall issue a permit for the sale thereof. Such devices may be sold by wholesalers regularly transacting business as such, but it shall be unlawful for any wholesaler to knowingly sell such devices to any unlicensed retailer.

(2) The offering for sale, distribution, or other disposition by means of a vending machine or other automatic machine of such devices is expressly prohibited.

(3) Any such vending machine or other automatic machine shall be destroyed when found in violation hereof. Possession of such devices by any unlicensed retailer in his place of business shall be prima facie evidence of sale.

(4) The State Board of Pharmacy shall enforce the terms of this section and may establish minimum standards of quality for such devices which standards of quality shall be such as will tend to reduce the likelihood of contracting a venereal disease.

(5) Any person who violates any of the provisions of this section or regulation of the Board shall be guilty of a misdemeanor."

The purely regulatory character of this legislation was emphasized in the case of Cavalier Vending Corp. v. State Board of Pharmacy, 195 Va. 626, app. dism'd, 347 U.S. 995. Prohibition of the sale of prophylactics by vending machine was held to be constitutional, whereas their sale through licensed retail outlets was justified as discouraging their improper use.

New Jersey, in effect, prohibits the sale of contraceptives by vending machine (the statute does not refer to them, but the courts have so construed the law). Title 2A (N.J. Stat. Ann. (Supp. 1955) states that:

"Any person who, without just cause, utters or exposes to the view of another, or possesses with intent to utter or expose to the view of another, or to sell the same, any instrument, medicine or other things, designed or purporting to be designed for the prevention of conception or the procuring of abortion, or who in any way advertises or aids in advertising the same, or in any manner, whether by recommendation for or against its use or otherwise, gives or causes to be given, or aids in giving any information how or where any instrument, medicine or other thing may be had, seen, bought or sold, is a disorderly person."

The owner of a prophylactic vending machine was held to be a "disorderly person" under this statute in State v. Tracy, 29 N.J. Super. 145 (App. Div. 1953), petition for certification denied, 15 N.J. 79 (1954). A similar result was reached in Sanitary Vendors Inc. v. Byrne, 72 N.J. Super. 276 (1962), aff'd 40 N.J. 157, which held the above statute to prohibit the sale of prophylactics by vending machine and for "illegal contraception" (not, however, including sales by druggists or dispensation by doctors "for uses not in connection with illegal conduct").

Other Laws

Washington law covers both contraception and prophylactics, as well as abortion. (All states, of course, have abortion laws, but only some mention the matter in connection with other statutes). The first pertinent statute appearing in the Washington laws is found in Section 9.68.030, Title 9, Chapter 9.68 (Wash. Rev. Stat. (1952) and contains the following provisions:

"Every person who shall expose for sale, loan or distribution any instrument or article, or any drug or medicine, for the prevention of conception, or for causing unlawful abortion; or shall write, print, distribute or exhibit any card, circular, pamphlet, advertisement or notice of any kind, stating when, where, how, or of whom such article or medicine can be obtained, shall be guilty of a misdemeanor."

The sections dealing with prophylactics are found in Title 18, Chapter 81 and are set forth below:

Section 18.81.010 provides a definition of prophylactic as "any device or medical preparation or compound which is or may be used, designed, intended or which has or may have special utility, for the prevention and/or treatment of venereal diseases."

Section 18.81.020 relates to the sale of prophylactics and provides that "It shall be unlawful for any person to sell any prophylactic at wholesale or retail without having, respectively, a valid and subsisting wholesale dealer's license issued under the provisions of this chapter; nor shall any licensed wholesale dealer make any sale other than at wholesale, nor any licensed retail dealer make any sale other than at retail."

Section 18.81.025 excepts physicians and surgeons from the requirements relating to sale in the following terms:

"It shall be unlawful for any person, except a physician and surgeon duly licensed as such under the laws of the state of Washington, to sell any prophylactic without being the holder of a valid and subsisting license issued under the provisions of this chapter or to sell any prophylactic except as authorized by the provisions of this chapter."

The conditions for eligibility to obtain a retailer's license are contained in Section 18.81.030 as follows:

"No retail dealer's license shall be issued to any person who does not hold a valid and subsisting license authorizing the holder to operate a pharmacy, nor shall any sale be made by any licentiate except in his place of business."

The sale of inefficacious prophylactics is prohibited under Section 18.81.060 by the provision that "No person shall sell any prophylactic which has no efficacy as an agent for the prevention and/or treatment of venereal diseases; and the action of the board in determining whether a particular prophylactic is or is not efficacious shall be conclusive, except for arbitrary, fraudulent or capricious action."

Later sections provide for seizure and destruction of

nonconforming prophylactics and prescribe the penalties for various violations.

In the case of State v. Northwest Drug Co., 15 Wash. 2d 634 (1942), a drug concern was held not guilty of selling as a wholesaler by selling two gross of prophylactics to a State Board of Pharmacy inspector, since the latter had no intention of reselling to users.

The Wyoming statutes governing contraception, abortion, and obscenity are quite comprehensive. The principal provisions appear in three sections of the statutes. The first of these relates to the sale, exhibition and advertising of "obscene, lewd or indecent articles or things" and provides as follows:

"Whoever sells or lends, or offers to sell or lend, or gives away, or in any manner exhibits, or has in his possession, with or without intent to sell, lend or give away, any obscene, lewd, indecent, or lascivious book, pamphlet, paper, drawing lithograph, engraving, picture, daguerreotype, photograph, stereoscopic picture model, cast, instrument or article of indecent or immoral use, or instrument or article for procuring abortion or for self-pollution, or medicine for procuring abortion, or preventing conception; or advertises the same or any of them for sale; or writes or prints any letter, circular, hand-bill, card, book, pamphlet, advertisement or notice of any kind; or gives information orally, stating when, how, where, or by what means, or of whom, any of the obscene, lewd, indecent, or lascivious articles or things hereinbefore mentioned, can be purchased, borrowed, presented, or otherwise obtained, or are manufactured; or manufactures, or draws and exposes or draws with intent to sell, or have sold, or prints any such articles or things shall be fined not more than one hundred dollars, to which may be added imprisonment in the county jail not more than six months; but nothing contained in this section, or in the next two sections * * * shall be construed to affect teaching in regular chartered medical colleges, or the publication of standard medical books, or the practice of regular practitioners of medicine or druggists in their legitimate business." (Wyoming Stat. Ann. (1957), Title 6,

Chapter 6, Section 6-103)

The following section of the statute (Section 6-104) pertains to the mailing, conveyance, or giving of oral information respecting similar matters. Its provisions are:

"Whoever deposits in any postoffice in this state, or places in charge of any person to be carried or conveyed, any lewd, obscene, indecent or lascivious book, paper, pamphlet, drawing, lithograph, engraving, picture, daguerreotype, photograph, (steroscopic) picture, model, cast, instrument or article of indecent or immoral use, or instrument or article for procuring abortion, or for self-pollution, or medicine for procuring abortion or preventing conception, or any circular or hand-bill, card, advertisement, book, pamphlet, or notice of any kind; or gives oral information, stating when, where, how, or of whom such articles or things or any of them can be purchased or otherwise obtained: or knowingly carries, or conveys the same, except in the United States mail, shall be fined not more than one hundred dollars, to which may be added imprisonment in the county jail not more than six months."

The final section (Section 6-105) deals primarily with publication and advertising as follows:

"Whoever prints or publishes any advertisement of any secret drug or nostrum purporting to be for the exclusive use of females or which cautions females against their use when in a condition of pregnancy; or in any way publishes any account or description of any drug, medicine, instrument, or apparatus for preventing conception, or for procuring abortion or miscarriage; or sells or gives away, or keeps for sale or gratuitous distribution, any newspaper, circular, pamphlet, or book containing such advertisement, account or description, or any secret drug or nostrum purporting to be exclusively for the use of females, or for preventing conception, or procuring abortion or miscarriage, shall be fined not more than one hundred dollars, to which may be added imprisonment in the county jail not more than six months."

Constitutional Challenge to State Contraceptive Laws

In June, 1977, the U.S. Supreme Court struck down the New York Statute which prohibited the sale or distribution of nonprescription contraceptives to minors under 16. The Court held that "the right of privacy in connection with decisions affecting procreation extends to minors as well as to adults" and that the restriction burdened minors' access to contraceptives without serving any significant state interest. This was the first time the Supreme Court had considered minors' rights to contraception.

The Court held further that the provision of the law restricting the distribution of nonprescription contraceptives to persons over 16 to licensed pharmacists was an undue burden on the individual's constitutional right to decide whether to bear a child.

In addition, the Court invalidated the law's prohibition on advertising and display of contraceptives. The ruling applies to advertising and display of prescription as well as nonprescription contraceptives, at least when the advertising is by persons licensed to sell such products.

With respect to the limitation on sale of nonprescription contraceptives to persons over 16 and the ban on advertising and display, the Court reasoned that state regulations which infringe on constitutional rights of privacy and free speech are valid only if they are supported by a compelling state interest. The Court held that New York failed to show such an interest.

Responding to the state's argument that past Supreme Court decisions upholding the constitutional right to use contraceptives (the *Griswold v. Connecticut* case among others) did not establish a right of access to contraceptives, the Court said: "*Griswold* may no longer be read as holding only that a state may not prohibit a married couple's use of contraceptives. Read in the light of its progeny, the teaching of *Griswold* is that the Constitution protects individual decisions in matters of child-bearing from unjustified intrusion by the state. Restrictions on the distribution of contraceptives clearly burdens the freedom to make such decisions." The decision points out that a total ban on sale of contraceptives would interfere in decisions regarding procreation as harshly as a ban on their use and might have an "even more devastating" effect, since it could be more easily enforced than a ban on use.

The Court pointed out that following its decision in *Roe v. Wade*, which held that a woman has a constitutional right to abortion, the Court in *Doe v. Bolton, Planned Parenthood of Central Missouri v. Danforth*, and *Bigelow v. Virginia*, held unconstitutional state statutes that did not prohibit abortion altogether but limited, in a variety of ways, a woman's access to abortion. "The significance of these cases is that they establish that the same test must be applied to state regulations that burden an individuals right to decide to prevent contraception or terminate pregnancy by substantially limiting access to the means of effectuating that decision as is applied to state statutes that prohibit the decisions entirely." Both types of regulations, the Court said, can be justified only by a compelling state interest and must be narrowly drawn to reflect only those interests, because access to contraceptives is "essential to exercise of the constitutionally protected right of decision in matters of childbearing that is the underlying foundation of the holdings" in *Griswold, Baird* and *Roe*.

The ruling does not apply to restrictions on or prohibition of vending machine sales of contraceptives, which the Court expressly excluded from the scope of its decision.

Regulating Advertising

Relying chiefly on its decision the previous year in *Virginia State Board of Pharmacy v. Virginia Citizens Consumer Council*, which held that a state may not "completely suppress the dissemination of concededly truthful information about entirely lawful activity," even when the information could be categorized as "commercial speech," the Court ruled that the New York ban on advertising and display of contraceptives violated the First Amendment right of free speech by completely suppressing all information about the availability and price of contraceptives.

States Affected by Carey v. Population Services International.

Besides New York, 12 states carry laws restricting in some manner the sale or distribution of contraceptives: Arkansas, Idaho, Maryland, Massachusetts, Minnesota, Montana, Nebraska, New Jersey, North Dakota, Oregon, Texas, and Wisconsin.

The most common restrictions are limitations on who may sell or distribute contraceptives (usually limited to pharmicists, physicians, hospitals, clinics, and health agencies) and prohibition of vending machine sales of contraceptives.

In Maryland, Massachusetts and North Dakota, the only restriction on distribution of contraceptives is the prohibition of vending machine sales, and Maryland has some exceptions to that restriction. Arkansas, Idaho, Minnesota, Montana and Wisconsin prohibit vending machine sales in addition to regulating or restricting the sale of distribution of contraceptives in other respects. As interpreted by the courts, New Jersey law seems to restrict vending machine sales. Statutes which apply only to vending machine sales may be valid, since, again, the Supreme Court expressly excluded them from the scope of its ruling.

Nebraska's only restriction is on the sale or distribution of "any secret nostrum, drug or medicine for the purpose of preventing conception" or causing an abortion. Texas prohibits nonphysicians and nonpharmicists from selling contraceptives "on the streets or in other public places." Oregon has a statute providing for wholesale and manufacturing licenses for the sale of articles to prevent conception.

In addition to the states which regulate the sale and distribution of contraceptives, 11 states: Colorado, Hawaii, Idaho, Iowa, Kentucky, Michigan, Nebraska, Oregon, Texas, Utah and Washington — all regulate or restrict the sale of prophylactics, which they define as devices intended to prevent disease. Four states, Hawaii, Montana, North Dakota and South Dakota, prohibit vending machine sales of prophylactics.

Eleven states restrict or regulate the advertising of contraceptives: Arizona, Arkansas, Hawaii, Idaho, Indiana, Louisiana, Michigan, Montana, Nebraska, New Jersey and Wisconsin. Louisiana and Nebraska, however, restrict the advertising of only "secret" nostrums or drugs.

Seven states: California, Colorado (vending machines only), Idaho, Kentucky, Michigan, Nebraska and Utah, restrict or regulate the display of contraceptives.

The following states have laws restricting or regulating the advertising of prophylactics: Arkansas, California, Colorado, Hawaii, Idaho, Michigan, Montana, South Dakota, Utah, West Virginia and Wyoming.

No state has a provision similar to the New York prohibition on distribution of nonprescription contraceptives to minors under 16. Although parental consent for contraception was not a specific issue in the case, the Court's reasoning indicates that such a requirement with respect to nonprescription contraceptives would be an unconstitutional infringement of the minor's rights.

Exactly how and/or to what degree the various state laws will stand up in light of the *Carey* cannot be anticipated, but reader should be alert to their vulnerability to judicial challenge.

Chapter III
LEGAL STATUS OF ARTIFICIAL SEMINATION

The pertinence of the problem of artificial insemination to planned parenthood is obvious. It represents the converse of contraception and may be indicated by a number of conditions, the chief of which are infertility or impotence in the male, or the presence of hazardous eugenic considerations. There are three basic categories of artificial insemination: employment of the semen of the husband (A.I.H.), that of a third-party donor (A.I.D.) or a mixture of both (A.I.H.D.). The incidence of success of this technique is relatively encouraging, particularly in the case of A.I.D. Limitations on the successful employment of A.I.H. inheres in the fact that in most instances there is an existing seminal defect of some kind to begin with.

The legal status of artificial insemination is unclear for the simple reason that statutory law is virtually non-existent, and case law meager and conflicting. A.I.H., of course, presents relatively few legal complications, as the offspring are unquestionably legitimate. One potential problem is the possibility of divorce proceedings on the ground of nonconsummation, but this would ordinarily be confined to cases involing impotence. A.I.D., on the other hand, presents a host of potential legal problems, including adultery, legitimacy, inheritance, and so forth.

LEGALITY OF ARTIFICIAL INSEMINATION: The absence of any common law commentary on artificial insemination, because of the insignificant incidence of such procedures until late in the nineteenth century, together with the continued want of statute or definitive case precedent, renders the exact legal status of this practice highly speculative. Nevertheless the fact that it is nowhere legally prohibited by express legislation tends to favor at least a tentative conclusion that the procedure is legal. An even stronger indication is the relatively favorable concensus of judicial dicta and the fact that tacit recognition of its legality is inferrable, from the Sanitary Code of New York City which sets forth regulations governing the selection of A.I.D. donors. This does not mean, however, that the practice may not involve criminality under certain circumstances. This problem may, for example, arise in connection with alleged adultery. This issue could arise, of course, only in a jurisdiction where adultery is criminal. Assuming this, the next question is whether artificial insemination, involving a third-party donor, constitutes an adulterous act. The first recorded case dealing with this question was <u>Orford v. Orford</u>, 49 Ont. L. R. 15 (1921). After noting that previously no act other than actual intercourse had been regarded as adultery, the court went on to hold that the "essence of the offense of adultery consists not in the moral turpitude of the act of sexual intercourse, but in the voluntary surrender to another person of the reproductive powers or faculties of the guilty person and any submission of those powers to the services or enjoyment of any person other than the husband or wife comes within the definition of adultery." The court further held that the introduction of "the seed" of a third party by artificial insemination without the knowledge of the husband constituted adultery, disentitling the wife to alimony. The decision is devoid of any indication of whether the husband's consent might alter this conclusion. The first American case to consider this issue, <u>Hoch v. Hoch,</u> Cook Co., Ill. Cir. Ct. (1948) resulted in a diametrically opposed holding—namely that such artificial insemination was not adulterous. Further compounding the conflict, however, a subsequent Illinois case, <u>Doornboos v. Doornboos</u> (Super Ct. Cook Co., Ill. (1954) held that the practice of A.I.D. constituted adultery, whether with or without the consent of the husband. On the other hand, a 1958 Scottish case, <u>MacLennan v. MacLennan</u> (Sess. Cas. 105 (Scot.), reverts to the opposing position. In this case the court said:

"While the primary purpose of sexual intercourse is the

procreation, in the eyes of the law surrender of the reproductive organs is not necessary to consummate the act of intercourse. Expedients may be used by the parties to secure birth prevention or the woman may have previously undergone an operation by which her reproductive organs may have been removed, or they may have ceased to function from natural causes and yet the conjunction of the sexual organs involving at least some degree of penetration would constitute intercourse, and * * * adultery. * * * the law looks at the act and not at the result. * * * ."

While it is impossible to arrive at a categorical answer, the overall tenor of these decisions, as well as existing legal commentaries thereon would indicate that American appellate courts probably would consider artificial insemination as non-adulterous, but, as yet, there is no guiding precedent.

On the question of legitimacy of the offspring, there is likewise a paucity of precedent. In <u>Doornboos v. Doornboos,</u> 121 Ill. App. Ct. Rep., 473 (1956), the child was declared illegitimate, while two New York decisions reflect conflicting views. In Strnad v. Strnad, 78 N.Y.S. 2d 390 (1948), the court held that the child was legitimate if the husband consented to the A.I.D., on the theory that the situation paralleled that of legitimatization of a child by subsequent marriage of the parents. The parallel, of course, is not perfect, particularly in view of the disparate parentage. The more recent case of <u>Gursky v. Gursky,</u> 242 N.Y.S. 2d 406 resulted in a contrary holding, based on the following grounds:

(1) No New York statute dealt with the question.
(2) At common law, the child was "born out of wedlock" and hence illegitimate.
(3) A New York law defined one born out of wedlock as a child begotten and born "out of lawful matrimony".
(4) The absence of any other guiding precedent.

In any event, it seems improbable that either the physician or the wife submitting to the procedure would be guilty of adultery, or the former of rape, even if the act were performed without the latter's consent, although in this event the doctor would probably be civilly or criminally liable for battery.

FUTURE OF ARTIFICIAL INSEMINATION: The dearth of precedent and absence of pertinent legislation clearly indicate the need for appropriate legislative measures dealing with this practice. Even in jurisdictions like Illinois, where, on the basis of the Doornbos case, the child might be considered illegitimate, satisfactory proof of such status may be difficult. Children born in lawful wedlock are presumed to be legitimate, although this presumption is rebuttable (but only by convincing proof). In most states, however, testimony by either spouse respecting adultery or nonaccess is inadmissible, which would presumably preclude testimony confirming the alleged artificial insemination. As already noted, the only official regulation respecting artificial insemination currently in effect appears in the New York City Sanitary Code (Section 1,12), which provides that only duly licensed physicians may "collect, offer for sale, sell or give away human seminal fluid for the purpose of causing artificial insemination." The section also provides that donors must submit to a physical examination and be free from certain diseases and hereditary defects. The physician is required to keep a record showing his name, that of the recipient, result of the examination, and the date of the insemination. These records must remain confidential and available only to authorized individuals.

What follows are the few states which legislation dealing with artificial semination. As can be seen, these laws legitimize the child if both spouses signed consent forms to the insemination. No distinction appears to be made between husband and third party donors.

ARKANSAS STAT. 61-141 - Concerning the effect of illegitimacy on Interstate succession: ...(c) any child conceived following artificial insemination of a married woman with the consent of her husband shall be treated as their child for all purposes of Intestate succession; consent of the husband is presumed unless the contrary is shown by clear and convincing evidence.

CALIFORNIA PENAL CODE, TITLE 9, §270 - A father of either a legitimate or illegitimate minor child who willfully omits without lawful excuse to furnish necessary clothing, food, shelter or medical attendance or other remedial care for his child is guilty of a misdemeanor and punishable by a fine not exceeding one thousand dollars ($1,000) or by imprisonment in a county jail not exceeding one year, or by both such fine and imprisonment.... The husband of a woman who bears a child as a result of artificial insemination shall be considered the father of that child for the purposes of this section, if he consented in writing to the artificial insemination.

GEORGIA CODE §74-101.1 - (a) All children born within wedlock, or within the usual period of gestation thereafter, who have been conceived legitimate if both the husband and wife consent in writing to the use and administration of artificial insemination. (b) Physicians and surgeons licensed to practice medicine in accordance with and under the provisions of Chapter 84-9 shall be the only persons authorized to administer or perform artificial insemination upon any female human being. Any other person or persons who shall attempt to administer or perform, or who shall actually administer or perform, artificial insemination upon any female human being shall be guilty of a felony, and on conviction therefore shall be punished by imprisonment in the penitentiary for not less than one year nor more than five years. (c) Any physician or surgeon who shall obtain written authorization signed by both the husband and wife authorizing him to perform or administer artificial insemination shall be relieved of civil liability to the husband and wife or to any child conveived by artificial insemination for the result or results of said artificial insemination: Provided, however, the written authorization provided for herein shall not relieve any physician or surgeon from any civil liability arising from his or her own negligent administration or performance of artificial insemination.

KANSAS STATUTES §23-128 - The Technique of heterologous artificial insemination may be performed in this state at the request and with the consent in writing of the husband and wife desiring the utilization of such technique for the purpose of conceiving a child or children.

KANSAS STATUTES §23-129 - Any child or children heretofore or hereafter born as the result of heterologous artificial insemination shall be considered at law in all respects the same as a naturally conceived child of the husband and wife so requesting and consenting to the use of such technique.

KANSAS STATUTES §23-130 - After the effective date of this act the consent provided for in this act shall be executed and acknowledged by both the husband and wife and the person who is to perform the technique, and an original thereof may be filed under the same rules as adoption papers in the probate court of the county in which such husband and wife reside. The written consent so filed shall not be open to the general public, and the information contained therein may be released only to the persons executing such consent, or to persons having a legimate interest therein as evidenced by a specific court order.

OKLAHOMA STATUTES - ARTIFICIAL INSEMINATION
OKLAHOMA STAT. TIT. 10, §551 - The technique of heterologous artificial insemination may be performed in this State by persons duly authorized to practice medicine at the request and with the consent in writing of the husband and wife desiring the utilization of such technique for the purpose of conveiving a child or children.

OKLAHOMA STAT. TIT. 10 §552 - Any child or children born as the result thereof shall be considered at law in all respects the same as a naturally conveived legitimate child of the husband and wife so requesting and consenting to the use of such technique.

OKLAHOMA STAT. TIT. 10 §553 - No person shall perform the technique of heterologous artificial insemination unless currently licensed to practice medicine in this State, and then only at the request and with the written consent of the husband and wife desiring the utilization of such technique. The said consent shall be executed and acknowledged by both the husband and wife and the person who is to perform the technique, and the judge having jurisdiction over the adoption of children, and an original thereof shall be filed under the same rules as adoption papers. The written consent so filed shall not be open to the general public, and the information contained therein may be released only to the persons executing such consent, or to persons having legitimate interest therein as evidenced by a specific court order.

NORTH CAROLINA GENERAL STATUTES, SECTION 49A-1 - Any child or children born as the result of heterologous artificial insemination shall be considered at law in all respects the same as a naturally conceived legitimate child of the husband and wife requesting and consenting in writing to the use of such technique. (1971, c. 260)

Chapter IV
STERILIZATION AND THE LAW

Sterilization, the surgical inducement of sterility, may be subdivided into three general categories: eugenical, therapeutic, and contraceptive. Eugenical sterilization, sanctioned by statute in 28 jurisdictions, is designed to prevent the propagation of defective, and, sometimes, criminal classes of individuals on the now dubious doctrine—excepting a very restricted class of mental disorders—that such proclivities are inheritable or follow medelian ratios. Even assuming the premise, the efficacy of eugenical sterilization would be extremely low since it would not apply to "carriers" who greatly outnumber "defectives," yet possess the same potentiality for propagation. Eugenical sterilization is commonly a compulsory procedure if the statutes are taken literally, but in actual practice the majority of such operations are undertaken as a result of a request by either the patient or his family. Three states—California, Iowa, and Michigan—prescribe an alternative procedure whereunder the patient or his guardian agrees to the operation which is then ordered by judicial or administrative authorities. In Minnesota and Vermont, the latter method of proceeding is exclusive.

Therapeutic sterilization is rarely, if ever, expressly prescribed by statute, but its legality is implicit in a provision commonly found in eugenical sterilization statutes that nothing therein may be "construed to prevent the medical or surgical treatment for sound therapeutic reasons." In any case, it is virtually certain that therapeutic sterilization is permissible solely on a voluntary basis.

Sexual sterilization designed to prevent conception is, in selective circumstances, an invaluable contraceptive technique, of unimpeachable scientific validity, yet there is a remarkable paucity of precedent, statutory or judicial, defining its legal status. It is indicated chiefly in cases of multiparity, and is the surest, cheapest technique which, incidentally, interferes least with consummation of the sexual act. Nevertheless a number of elements militate against its indiscriminate employment. Foremost, of course, is the absolute opposition of the Catholic Church, as exemplified in an address by Pope Pius XII in 1951 in which the Pontiff said: "Direct sterilization, that which aims at making procreation impossible both as a means and an end, is a grave violation of the moral law, and therefore illicit. Even public authority has no right to permit it under the pretext of any indication whatsoever, and still less to prescribe it * * * ." Another restraining factor is the relative finality of the operation. Scientific estimates of the possibility of surgical reversal vary widely from extremely low to as high as 50%, but there is no doubt that reversibility is attainable in a considerable number of instances. Sometimes it occurs spontaneously through "recanalization" — reunion of the cut tubes—but, of course, this type of reversal is unwelcome. Recanalization occurs most frequently in vasectomy, and it is also probable that surgical reversal is more likely to succeed in the male.

Vasectomy consists of cutting the vas deferens, which connects the testes and the urinary canal, thus preventing sperm from passing into the latter. It requires several weeks for sterility to ensue with certainty, since sperm present prior to the operation may still be ejaculated. Vasectomy is by far the simpler of the two principal sterilization procedures (and the only one in the case of the male), and is ordinarily performed in the physician's office under a local anesthetic. In the female, while there are several possible procedures, the one almost invariably employed for contraceptive purposes is known as tubal ligation or salpingectomy. This consists of cutting the fallopian tubes and tying off the separate ends. It is performed in a hospital under general anesthesia and constitutes major surgery.

A final precautionary consideration relates to the possibility of adverse psychological reactions or reduced capacities for sexual satisfaction. Research reveals, however, that the incidence of such sequalae is very low. It is, however, a possibility which cannot be entirely ignored and may, in certain instances, be serious. There is also the possibility that a request for sterilization may actually constitute an unconscious desire for self-mutilation.

LEGAL STATUS OF CONTRACEPTIVE STERILIZATION: The legal position of voluntary contraceptive sterilization appears in most jurisdictions to be an open question, due to the absence of pertinent legislation or binding precedent. Although, as already noted, 28 states have eugenical sterilization laws, such statutes cast little, if any, light on the status of sexual sterilization for contraceptive purposes.

It seems clear that, at common law, voluntary *therapeutic* sterilization must be regarded as legal, which probably accounts for the provisos appearing in many eugenical statutes (known as "saving clauses") which, as has been observed, exclude any construction which would prevent medical or surgical treatment for "sound therapeutic reasons".

Compulsory sterilization, on the other hand, whether therapeutic or eugenical, is undoubtedly unlawful in the absence of authorizing statute. North Carolina is among those jurisdictions which permits the sterilization of the mentally ill and retarded on a compulsory basis on the part of state social service agencies. In a 1976 North Carolina Supreme Court case, *In Re Sterilization of Joseph Lee Moore*, the North Carolina statute was upheld as constitutional. The case as a whole, reviews the various legal and moral dimensions of compulsory sterilization and it is useful to produce here a substantial part of that decision for the purpose of giving the reader what will continue to be the legal status of his increasingly important subject in the law of sterilization and family planning:

SUPREME COURT OF NORTH CAROLINA
IN RE STERILIZATION OF JOSEPH LEE MOORE

On 21 May 1975 a petition was filed in Forsyth County District Court by Gerald M. Thornton, Director, Forsyth County Department of Social Services, requesting that the court enter an order authorizing the sterilization of Joseph Lee Moore, a minor. The petition was accompanied by the consent of the respondent, Joseph Lee Moore; and his mother, Dora I. Moore. A psychological report included in the petition indicated that Joseph is presently functioning at a moderately retarded level of measured intelligence, with a Full Scale I.Q. of under 40 and a Test Age score of 8. The petitioner believed Joseph to be a proper subject for sterilization because it is likely that unless sterilized he would procreate a child or children who would probably have serious physical, mental or nervous diseases or deficiencies. The accompanying statement by the examining physician, Dr. Ruth O'Neal found no known contraindication to the requested surgical procedure.

The respondent, through his guardian ad litem and attorney, in apt time objected to the petition and requested a hearing. This matter was heard on 29 July 1975 before A. Lincoln Sherk, Jr., in Forsyth District Court, Juvenile Division. The respondent filed a mortion to quash and dismiss the petition, alleging that G.S. 35-36, et seq., was unconstitutional. This motion was allowed and notice of appeal was given by the State to Forsyth Superior Court.

The matter was heard de novo before McConnell, J., at the 28 July 1975 Civil Session of Forsyth Superior Court. The respondent again made his motion to quash or dismiss the petition. Judge McConnell allowed the motion, finding G.S. 35-36 through G.S. 35-50, inclusive, unconstitutional. The District Attorney for the Twenty-first Judicial District excepted to the judgement and for the state gave notice of appeal to the Court of Appeals. The respondent petitioned the Supreme Court to hear this matter prior to determination by the Court of Appeals. This petition was allowed on 27 August 1975.

MOORE, Justice.

The only question before us on this appeal is the constitutionality of G.S. 35-36 through G.S. 35-50, inclusive.

The respondent attacks these statutes on the grounds that they are violative of the Due Process Clause of the Fourteenth Amendment to the United States Constitution and the Law of the Land Clause of Article I, Section 19, of the North Carolina Constitution, both from procedural and substantive standpoints, that they deny the respondent equal protection of the law, are unconstitutionally vague and arbitrary, and provide for cruel and unusual punishment. The term "law of the land" as used in Article I, Section 19, of the Constitution of North Carolina, is synonymous with "due process of law" as used in the Fourteenth Amendment to the Federal Constitution.

The right of a state to sterilize retarded or insane persons was first upheld by the United States Supreme Court in Buck v. Bell, 274 U.S. 200, 47 S.Ct. 584, 71 L.Ed. 1000 (1927). In that case, in upholding a Virginia sterilization law, the Court held that the site may provide for the sterilization of a feebleminded inmate of a state institution where it is found that she is the probable potential parent of socially inadequate offspring likewise afflicted, and that she may be sterilized without detriment to her general health, and that her welfare and that of society will be promoted by her sterilization. Since Buck, many states have passed sterilization laws.

Most of these statutes have been declared constitutional. The grounds for declaring some of the statutes unconstitutional were lack of notice and a hearing, In Re Hendrickson, 12 Wash. 2d 600, 123 P.2d 322 (1942), In Re Opinion of the Justices, 230 Ala. 543, 162 So. 123 (1935), Williams v. Smith, 190 Ind. 526, 131 N.E. 2 (1921); equal protection because limited to those imprisoned or committed, or cruel and unusual punishment.

Our research does not disclose any case which holds that a state does not have the right to sterilize an insane or a retarded person if notice and hearing are provided, if it is applied equally to all persons, and if it is not prescribed as a punishment for a crime.

Respondent contends, however, that not all the requirements of procedural due process have been met in this case. A former sterilization statute was held unconstitutional by this Court on procedural grounds, specifically that notice and a hearing were not provided. The present statute, effective 1 January 1975, sought to correct the defects found in the former statute. G.S. 35-36 and G.S. 35-37 both provided that "no operation authorized in this section shall be lawful unless and until the provisions of this Article shall first be complied with." G.S. 35-41 provides that at least twenty days prior to a hearing on the petition in the district court, a copy of such petition must be served on the resident of the institution, patient, or noninstitutional individual and on the legal or natural guardian, guardian ad litem, or next of kin of the resident of the institution, patient or noninstitutional individual. G.S. 35-44 provides for a hearing, if requested, before the judge of the district court. G.S. 35-44 also provides for an appeal from the judgement of the district court to the superior court for a trial de novo with the right upon the application of either party to be heard before a jury and the further right of appeal to the appellate courts for judicial review.

Despite the above specified safeguards, respondent still asserts that two important procedural rights have been omitted: (1) a provision that the State will provide the funds necessary to obtain a medical expert on behalf of the respondent and (2) the right of cross-examination. It is true that this statute does not require the State to pay a medical expert on behalf of the respondent. However, G.S. 7A-454 allows the court in its discretion to approve a fee for the services of an expert witness who testifies for an indigent person. We know of no constitutional mandate that requires more.

The right of cross-examination is specifically provided by G.S. 35-43.

We hold that the provisions of this statute far exceed the minimum requirements of procedural due process.

Respondent further contends that the statutes in question deny him substantive due process. "Due process" has a dual significance, as it pertains to procedure and a substantive law. As to procedure, it means notice and an opportunity to be heard and to defend in an orderly proceeding adapted to the nature of the case before a competent and impartial tribunal having jurisdiction of the cause. In substantive law, due process may be characterized as a standard of reasonableness and as such it is a limitation upon the exercise of the police power. "Undoubtedly, the State possesses the police power in its capacity as a sovereign, and in the exercise thereof, the legislature may enact laws, within constitutional limits, to protect or promote the health, morals, order, safety, and general welfare of society. (Citations omitted.)" State v. Ballance, 229 N.C. 764, 769, 51 S.E. 2d 730, 734 (1949). ". . . 'If a statute is to be sustained as a legitimate exercise of the police power, it must have a rational, real, or substantial relation to the public health, morals, order, or safety, or the general welfare'. . ."

The traditional substantive due process test has been that a statute must have a rational relation to a valid state objective. In a growing series of decisions, the United States Supreme Court has recognized a right of privacy emanating from the Fourteenth Amendment's concept of personal liberty or encompassed within the penumbra of the Bill of Rights that includes the abortion decision, Roe v. Wade, 410 U.S. 113, 93 S.Ct. 705, 35 L.Ed. 2d 147 (1973); certain marital activities, Loving v. Virginia, 388 U.S. 1, 87 S.Ct. 1817, 18 L.Ed. 2d 1010 (1967), and Griswold v. Connecticut, 381 U.S. 479, 85 S.Ct. 1678, 14 L.Ed. 2d 510 (1964); and procreation, Eisenstadt v. Baird, 405 U.S. 438, 92 S.Ct. 1029, 31 L.Ed. 2d 349 (1972), and Skinner v. Oklahoma, supra. In Eisenstadt, the Court specifically recognized ". . . the right of the individual, married or single, to be free from unwarranted governmental intrusion into matters so fundamentally affecting a person as the decision whether to bear or beget a child. . . ." However, in Roe v. Wade, supra, 410 U.S. at 154-55; 93 S.Ct. at 727, Mr. Justice Blackmun, speaking for the court, said:

". . . The Court's decisions recognizing a right of privacy also acknowledge that some state regulation in areas protected by that right is appropriate. As noted above, a State may properly assert important interests in safeguarding health, in maintaining medical standards, and in protecting potential life. . . .

"We therefore, conclude that the right of personal privacy . . . is not unqualified and must be considered against important state interests in regulation.

* * * * * *

"Where certain 'fundamental rights' are involved, the Court has held that regulation limiting these rights may be justified only by a 'compelling state interest', (citations omitted), prevent the normal sex drive of the person, it only prevents procreation. Therefore, the State may only be providing for the welfare of the individual when this individual is unable to do so for himself.

We hold that the sterilization of mentally ill or retarded persons under the safeguards as set out in G.S. 35-36 through G.S. 35-50, inclusive, is a valid and reasonable exercise of the police power, see Buck v. Bell, supra; Brewer v. Valk, supra, and that these state interests rise to the level of a compelling state interest.

The object of G.S. 35-36 through G.S. 35-50, inclusive, is to prevent the procreation of children by a mentally ill or retarded individual who because of physical, mental or nervous disease or deficiency which is not likely to materially improve, would probably be unable to care for a child or children or who would likely, unless sterilized, procreate a child or children who probably have serious physical, mental or nervous diseases or deficiencies. Considering this object, the classification under these statutes is reasonable.

Sterilization laws in several states have been declared unconstitutional because they affect only a certain class of mentally ill or retarded persons. Haynes v. Lapeer, Circuit Judge, supra; In Re Thompson, supra; Smith v. Board of Examiners of Feeble-Minded, supra. These cases declared laws unconstitutional when the law provided for a group of the feebleminded to be sterilized, such as those institutionalized, and for another group of feebleminded, such as those not institutionalized, not to be sterilized. G.S. 35-36 and G.S. 35-37 provide for the sterilization of all mentally ill or retarded persons inside or outside an institution who meet the requirements of these statutes. We have found no case that holds that sterilization of all mentally ill or retarded persons denies equal protection. Many cases have held otherwise. Buck v. Bell, supra; Smith v. Command, 231 Mich. 409, 204 N.W. 140 (1925). As said by Mr. Justice Holmes in Buck v. Bell, supra:

"But, it is said, however it might be if this reasoning were applied generally, it fails when it is confined to the small number who are in the institutions named and is not applied to the multitudes outside. It is the usual last resort of constitutional arguments to point out shortcomings of this sort. But the answer and that legislative enactments must be narrowly drawn to express only the legitimate state interests at stake. (citations omitted.)"

The right to procreate is not absolute but is vulnerable to a certain degree of state regulation. Roe v. Wade, supra; Buck v. Bell, supra. The two state interests recognized as paramount to the individual's freedom of choice in Roe v. Wade, supra, at least after the first trimester of pregnancy, were the state's concern with the health of the mother and the potential life of the child. The welfare of the parent and the future life and health of the unborn child are also the chief concerns of the State of North Carolina in authorizing sterilization of individuals under certain circumstances.

The interest of the unborn child is sufficient to warrant sterilization of a retarded individual. "The state's concern for the welfare of its citizenry extends to future generations and when there is overwhelming evidence. . . that a potential parent will be unable to provide a proper environment for a child becuase of his own mental illness or mental retardation, the state has sufficient interest to order sterilization." Cook v. State, 9 Or. App. 224, 495 P. 2d 768 (1972). The people of North Carolina also have a right to prevent the procreation of children who will become a burden on the State.. . . The United States Supreme Court has also held that the welfare of all citizens should take precedence over the rights of individuals to procreate. In Buck v. Bell, supra, the Court said: ". . . It is better for all the world, if instead of waiting to execute degenerate offspring for crime, or to let them starve for their imbecility, society can prevent those who are manifestly unfit from continuing their kind. The principle that sustains compulsory vaccination is broad enough to cover cutting the Fallopian tubes."

Furthermore, the sterilization of a mentally ill or retarded individual at certain times may be in the best interest of that individual. The mentally ill or retarded individual may not be capable of determining his inability to cope with children. In addition, he may be capable of functioning in society and caring for his own needs but may be unable to handle the additional responsibility of children. This individual also may not be able to practice other forms of birth control and therefore sterilization is the only available remedy. Sterilization itself does not is that the law does all that is needed when it does all that it can, indicates a policy, applies to all within the lines, and seeks to bring within the lines all similarly situated so far and so fast as its means allow. Of course so far as the operations enable those who otherwise must be kept confined to be returned to the world, and thus open the asylum to others, the equality aimed at will be more nearly reached."

Since the North Carolina law applies to all those named in the statute (G.S. 35-43), these statutes, G.S. 35-36 through G.S. 35-50, inclusive, do not violate the equal protection clauses of the United States Constitution or the Constitution of North Carolina.

Respondent next asserts that this legislation provides no adequate judicial standard to guide the court in reaching a decision whether to authorize the sterilization of an individual. Respondent points to the indefiniteness of the terms found in G.S. 35-43:

". . . If the judge of the district court shall find from the evidence that the person alleged to be subject to this section is subject to it and that because of a physical, mental, or nervous disease or deficiency which is not likely to materially improve, the person would probably be unable to care for a child or children; or, because the person would be likely, unless sterilized, to procreate a child or children which probably would have serious physical, mental, or nervous diseases or deficiencies, he shall enter an order and judgement authorizing the physician or surgeon named in the petition to perform the operation." (Emphasis added.)

Defendant contends that these indefinite terms render the statute unconstitutionally vague and arbitrary; that there exists no standard at all, except the subjective determination of an individual judge.

Several recent United States Supreme Court opinions have spoken to this issue of unconstitutional vagueness of lack of any judicial standard. In Parker v. Levy, 417 U.S. 733, 94 S.Ct. 2547, 41 L.Ed. 2d 439 (1974), the Court upheld the statute providing for court-martial of an officer for "conduct unbecoming an officer and a gentleman," against attack that it was too vague and arbitrary, stating, "'(t)he doctrine incorporates notions of fair notice or warning. Moreover, it requires legislatures to set reasonably clear guidelines for law enforcement officials and triers of fact in order to prevent "arbitrary and discriminatory enforcement." . . .' (Citation omitted.)" The same result was reached in Arnett v. Kennedy, 416 U.S. 134, 94, S.Ct. 1633, 40 L.Ed. 2d 15 (1974), where the Court sustained a statute providing for removal of nonprobationary federal employees only "for such cause as will promote the efficiency of the service." The Supreme Court has recognized that ". . . words inevitably contain germs of uncertainty and . . . there may be disputes about the meaning of such terms. . . .," but has reiterated that if they can be sufficiently understood and complied with, the statute will be upheld.

In the light of the foregoing principals, we believe that G.S. 35-36 through G.S. 35-50 meet this constitutional standard. The definitions of "mental disease," "mental illness" and "mental defective" are found in G.S. 35-1.1, the same chapter as the sterilization procedure, and are capable of being understood and complied with by the triers of fact with the help of experts in the field. It is conceded that the words "likely" and "probably" necessarily contain germs of uncertainty. However, it is the duty of the court to construe a statute, ambiguous in its meaning, so as to give effect to the legislative intent. Hobbs v. Moore County, supra. Here it is clear that the General Assembly intended to provide the mentally ill and defective with sufficient safeguards to prevent misuse of this potentially dangerous procedure. The statute does not specify the burden of proof that the petitioner must meet before the order authorizing the sterilization can be entered. In keeping with the intent of the General Assembly, clearly expressed throughout the article, that the rights of the individual must be fully protected, we hold that the evidence must be clear, strong and convincing before such an order may be entered. So construed, we hold that G.S. 35-36 through G.S. 35-50, inclusive, provide a sufficient judicial standard and are not unconstitutionally vague or arbitrary.

The respondent's next contention that sterilization amounts to cruel and unusual punishment is without basis in law in this case. The cruel and unusual punishment clause of the Constitution refers to those persons convicted of a crime. Since this is not a criminal proceeding, there is no basis for the cruel and unusual argument. The two cases cited in the amicus curiae brief, Davis v.

Berry, supra, and Mickle v. Henrichs, 262 F. 687 (D. Nev. 1918), both held that sterilization of criminals as part of a sentence upon conviction was cruel and unusual punishment. That question is not presented in this case and those cases are not pertinent to decision here.

This unfortunate respondent and his mother both consented to the performance of a vasectomy. While we do not attach much inportance to the respondent's consent due to his mental condition, his mother unquestionably is in a position to know what is best for the future of her child. Under the provisions of G.S. 35-36 through G.S. 35-50, inclusive, the rights of respondent and the state will be fully protected at hearing.

We hold, therefore, that the trial court erred in declaring these statutes unconstitutional. The judgement so entered is reversed.

Reversed.

APPENDICES

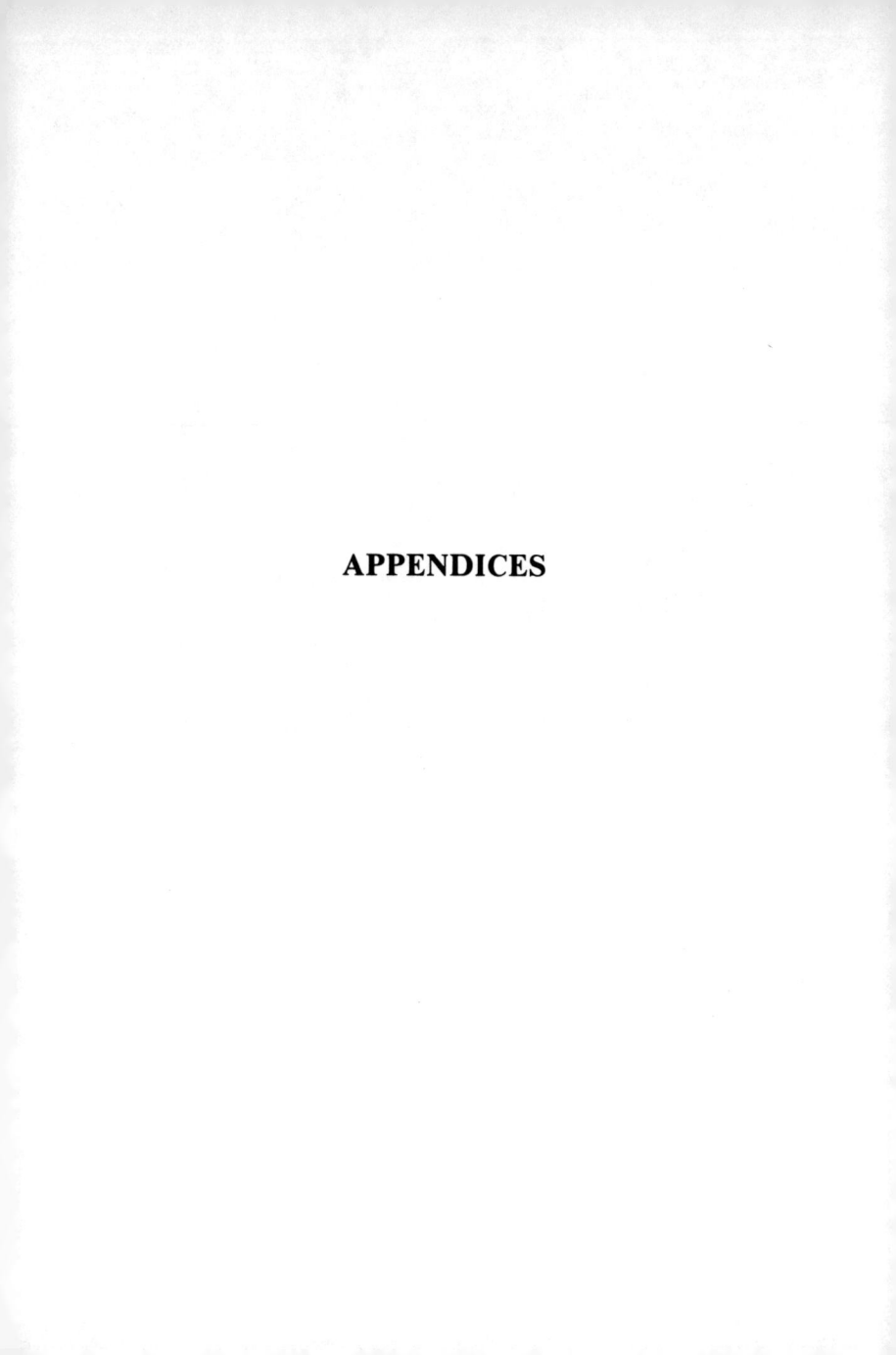

APPENDIX A

AMERICAN LAW INSTITUTE
MODEL PENAL CODE

Section 230.3. Abortion.

(1) <u>Unjustified Abortion</u>. A person who purposely and unjustifiably terminates the preganancy of another otherwise than by a live birth commits a felony of the third degree or, where the pregnancy has continued beyond the twenty-sixth week, a felony of the second degree.

(2) <u>Justifiable Aboration</u>. A licensed physician is justified in terminating a pregnancy if he believes there is substantial risk that continuance of the pregnancy would gravely impair the physical or mental health of the mother or that the child would be born with grave physical or mental defect, or that the pregnancy resulted from rape, incest, or other felonious intercourse. All illicit intercourse with a girl below the age of 16 shall be deemed felonious for purposes of this subsection. Justifiable abortions shall be performed only in a licensed hospital except in case of emergency when hospital facilities are unavailable. (Additional exceptions from the requirement of hospitalization may be incorporated here to take account of situations in sparsely settled areas where hospitals are not generally accessible.)

(3) <u>Physicians' Certificates; Presumption from Non-Compliance</u>. No abortion shall be performed unless two physicians, one of whom may be the person performing the abortion, shall have certified in writing the circumstances which they believe to justify the abortion. Such certificate shall be submitted before the abortion to the hospital where it is to be performed and in the case of abortion following felonious intercourse, to the prosecuting attorney or the police. Failure to comply with any of the requirements of this Subsection gives rise to a presumption that the abortion was justified.

(4) <u>Self-Abortion</u>. A woman whose pregnancy has continued beyond the twenty-sixth week commits a felony of the third degree if she purposely terminates her own pregnancy otherwise than by a live birth, or if she uses instruments, drugs or violence upon herself for that purpose. Except as justified under Subsection (2), a person who induces or knowingly aids a woman to use instruments,

drugs or violence upon herself for the purpose of terminating her pregnancy otherwise than by a live birth commits a felony of the third degree whether or not the pregnancy has continued beyond the twenty-sixth week.

(5) <u>Pretended Abortion</u>. A person commits a felony of the third degree if, representing that it is his purpose to perform an abortion, he does not act adapted to cause abortion in a pregnant woman although the woman is in fact not pregnant, or the actor does not believe she is. A person charged with unjustified abortion under Subsection (1) or an attempt to commit that offense may be convicted thereof upon proof of conduct prohibited by this Subsection.

(6) <u>Distribution of Abortifacients.</u> A person who sells, offers to sell, possesses with intent to sell, advertises, or displays for sale anything specially designed to terminate a pregnancy, or held out by the actor as useful for that purpose, commits a misdemeanor, unless:

(a) the sale, offer or display is to a physician or druggist or to an intermediary in a chain of distribution to physicians or druggists; or

(b) the sale is made upon prescription or order of a physician; or

(c) the possession is with intent to sell as authorized in paragraphs (a) and (b); or

(d) the advertising is addressed to persons named in paragraph (a) and confined to trade or professional channels not likely to reach the general public.

(7) <u>Section Inapplicable to Prevention of Pregnancy</u>. Nothing in this Section shall be deemed applicable to the prescription, administration or distribution of drugs or other substances for avoiding pregnancy, whether by preventing implanatation of a fertilized ovum or by any other method that operates before, at or immediately after fertilization.

APPENDIX B*

Summary and Analysis of State Laws Relating to Contraception

General Status of Laws Relating to Contraception

Since the mid-1960s there has been a veritable revolution in state laws relating to family planning services, and the sale, distribution and dissemination of information (including advertising and display) about contraceptives.

Whereas the history of state laws concerning birth control prior to that time had been dominated by restrictions and prohibitions patterned on the late nineteenth century 'Comstock Laws' (See Federal Laws and Policies Section, above), the trend since the mid-1960s has been to affirm state support of freer access to voluntary family planning information and services, and to establish family planning programs for state residents.

Almost half the states which had restrictive laws before the mid-1960s—16 states in all—have since repealed or liberalized their restrictive laws.[1] Eighteen states[2] and the District of Columbia adopted legislation authorizing state agencies to administer family planning programs. In a total of 28 states[3] —including 12 of the states with laws authorizing family planning programs—there is no statute at present restricting in any way the dissemination of information about, or the sale or distribution of, contraceptives to any person.

Of the remaining 22 states with some restrictions, three states—Louisiana, Nebraska and Pennsylvania —only prohibit the sale or advertising of "secret" drugs or nostrums to prevent conception, but since marketed contraceptives are hardly "secret," these statutes would appear to have little or no effect; Maine's only prohibition is against refilling prescriptions for oral contraceptives "from a copy of the original prescription"; Maryland and North Dakota prohibit vending machine sales of contraceptives only; Texas forbids sales of contraceptives "on streets and public places" by persons other than doctors or pharmacists; New Jersey prohibits the sale, advertising or display of contraceptives "without just cause," a statute which has been interpreted liberally by the courts. Most of the other laws regulate who may sell or distribute contraceptives (most often limited to pharmacists, physicians, hospitals, clinics and health agencies), or where and how they may be advertised or displayed. New York prohibits the sale of contraceptives to persons younger than 16, but this restriction does not apply to physicians. Wisconsin has a statute which forbids the sale or distribution of contraceptives to persons who are not married. Massachusetts had a similar provision in its statute which was declared unconstitutional by the United States Supreme Court (see discussion, below). Only three states—Indiana, South Dakota and Wisconsin—expressly forbid all dissemination of information about contraception, but these statutes are apparently subject to exceptions in practice and are not enforced generally; if they were, they would probably be subject to attack on First Amendment grounds.

The Griswold Case

Prior to 1965 many states had 'little Comstock laws' prohibiting or placing restrictions on the sale, advertising or display of "articles for the prevention of conception." Only Connecticut had a law actually prohibiting the *use* of contraceptives. In 1965, the United States Supreme Court in the *Griswold*[4] case recognized the right of married persons to practice birth control. In a case challenging the constitutionality of the Connecticut statute which forbade the use of contraceptives, the court held the statute to be violative of the right of marital privacy and, therefore, unconstitutional. Subsequently the case has been considered authority for the proposition that there is a right of privacy in matters relating to marriage, sex and the family. Since the *Griswold* decision at least 13[5] states have repealed or substantially liberalized their anticontraception laws. In this respect the *Griswold* case may be considered a bench mark, dividing an era dominated by laws restricting the availability of contraception from the era which actually encourages convenient access to and availability of family planning services.

Affirmative Laws

Of the 18 states which had affirmative family planning laws as of September 1, 1971, 10 had no statutory restrictions as to which residents of the state should be served by the state-administered programs authorized by the statutes[6]; seven set up programs for indigent persons only (usually welfare clients),[7] and three (California, Oklahoma and Ore-

---

*Source: Report of the National Center for Family Planning Services
Health Services and Mental Health Administration, U.S. Department of Health, Education and Welfare

gon) had separate provisions covering indigent persons and all others.

Most of these 18 states have laws which call for programs providing a full range of medical family planning services, supplies and information. Four state statutes call for information and/or referral services only. Alaska calls for information only for "all persons"; California's law, while calling for the provision of full family planning services for indigent persons, permits only information and referral for persons who are not indigent. California also provides that all marriage license applicants be provided a list of family planning clinics in their county. Illinois permits referral for indigent persons only. Hawaii provides for information only for marriage license applicants. In all these states, however, the extent of the actual programs carried out under these statutes is determined in large part by the availability of funds.

Many of the family planning programs authorized by these affirmative laws are, in general, quite comprehensive. The Tennessee statute,[8] for example, authorizes making medically acceptable contraceptive procedures, supplies and information readily and practicably available to persons desiring them regardless of sex, race, age, income, marital status, number of children, citizenship or motive. Colorado has a similar statute.[9] Both statutes provide that services shall be conditioned on "the availability of funds."

Oklahoma[10] and Kansas[11] authorize their state departments of health to establish family planning centers to furnish and disseminate information, means and methods of "planned parenthood" (Kansas), and to carry out clinical activities incident to child-spacing including medical examination, insertions of contraceptive devices and prescriptions of drugs (Oklahoma).

The significance of these affirmative family planning laws is that, despite the fact that a state may have no laws against furnishing family planning services, many people still lack access to effective means of controlling their fertility. This may be because they cannot afford to purchase family planning services from private physicians; they may lack information about what are the most effective methods; there may be no facility providing family planning services located conveniently to them; their physicians may have religious or other conscientious objections to providing them with contraceptives, or they may be deterred from seeking service if they are minors or unmarried because of fear of censure from their physicians or families. Government-subsidized family planning services are essential for these groups and others who have similar access difficulties and who might otherwise be subjected to unwanted pregnancy and childbearing.

Laws Relating to Sale and Distribution of Contraceptives

As of September 1971, there were 34 states[12] in which there was no law restricting or regulating[13] the sale or distribution of contraceptives.[14] The number of states with no laws on contraception has been increasing steadily since 1965 and the clear trend is toward the removal of all such barriers to the sale and distribution of contraceptives.[14a]

Statutory restrictions in the 16 remaining states vary from licensing requirements for those who may sell contraceptives, to limitations on distribution by certain categories of persons, to outright prohibitions against distribution of contraceptives by vending machines.[15]

Three states[16] have no restrictions on sale or distribution other than prohibiting the sale of contraceptives by vending machines. One state, Maryland, makes an exception, permitting sale by vending machine in certain places where alcoholic beverages are sold for consumption on the premises.[17] Maine forbids the selling of prescriptions for oral contraceptives "from a copy of the original prescription."[18] Twelve states[19] have statutes restricting or regulating the sale or distribution of contraceptives in other respects; of these, six[20] also expressly restrict sale of contraceptives by vending machine, and two, New Jersey and Iowa, restrict such vending machine sales by inference.[21]

Insofar as they restrict sale or distribution of contraceptives other than by vending machine, all of these state statutes (except Nebraska, see below) contain provisions exempting, or they have been construed to exempt, certain categories of persons (the most frequent being physicians, medical practitioners, and registered pharmacists) from the provisions of the statute. The result is that sale and distribution of contraceptives, at least by doctors and/or pharmacists, are legal in every state, although Wisconsin provides that sales and distribution can be made only to married persons.

Until recently, Massachusetts also provided that distribution of contraceptives could be made to married persons only. However, the Massachusetts statute, which permitted dispensation of "drugs and articles for use in birth control" only on a physician's prescription and only to married persons,[22] was held unconstitutional by the United States Supreme Court on March 22, 1972, in *Eisenstadt* v. *Baird*. 40 *U.S. Law Week* 4303 (March 21, 1972). A majority of the Court, in an opinion in which four justices joined, held that the statute's prohibition against the distribution of contraceptives except to married persons violated the rights of single persons under the Equal Protection Clause of the Fourteenth Amendment. Two justices, while joining in the result reached by the majority, wrote a separate opinion stating their view that the statutory requirement that contraceptives be dispensed only on a physician's prescription could not be sustained in the absence of proof that Emko Vaginal Foam, the contraceptive for the distribution of which Baird was convicted, was hazardous to health.

The Wisconsin statute makes it a misdemeanor to sell or dispose of contraceptives "to or for any unmarried person."[23] The United States Supreme Court decision in *Eisenstadt v. Baird,* supra, casts doubt on the validity of this provision.[24] (See State Profile, Wisconsin). For a discussion of restrictions relating to minors, see Summary and Analysis of State Laws Relating to Contraceptive Services to Minors, below.

Dissemination of Information, Advertising and Display

As of September, 1971, there were 33 states[25] in which no law restricted the dissemination of information (including advertising and display) about contraceptives. Three more states (Louisiana, Nebraska and Pennsylvania) had statutes restricting the advertising only of "secret" nostrums or drugs to prevent conception (See below). Of the remaining 14 states[26] with statutes containing some restriction on advertising, most have provisos exempting certain categories of advertisements from the statutory prohibitions; the most frequent permissible advertisements on contraceptives are those in medical and pharmaceutical publications, and those in "literature enclosed in and around the original package."[27]

Looking at display alone, as of the same date, there were 41 states[28] where no laws restricted the display of contraceptives. Of the remaining nine states[29] with restrictions, some, such as New Jersey[30] and Oregon[31] have liberalized the restrictions of the law by judicial interpretation, and in others, the State Attorney General has published opinions tending to limit the extent of the apparent restriction on display.[32]

Restrictions on the advertising, display or dissemination of information about contraceptives are sometimes challenged on First Amendment grounds.

For example, the Massachusetts statute prohibits exhibiting, advertising and circulating written information on contraceptives.[33] In *Baird v. Eisenstadt*[34] that part of the statute prohibiting the exhibition of contraceptives was held by the Massachusetts Supreme Court to be a violation of the First Amendment. Moreover, in an increasing number of cases, including *Griswold*, courts have recognized that the First Amendment protects the rights of those who wish to *receive* information, as well as the rights of those who wish to disseminate information.[35] It seems likely that within the near future, the validity of state statutes restricting advertising, display or dissemination of information on contraceptives will be resolved through a case which permits the courts to assess these issues.[36]

Limiting of the Scope of State Restrictive Statutes

Though many of the state statutes which regulate distribution or restrict advertising or display of contraceptives have language that seems quite broad, judicial interpretations and Attorneys General's opinions have tended to limit their scope. For example, in Arizona, a statute prohibiting advertising or giving any medicine or means for the prevention of conception[37] was construed to permit the dissemination of birth control information by a doctor to his patient or by Planned Parenthood. "Advertising" was limited to public commercial announcements advocating specific trade brands. *Planned Parenthood Committee of Phoenix, Inc. v. Maricopa County,* 92 Ariz. 231, 375 P. 2d 719 (1962).

In Iowa, where a statute prohibits the advertising, sale or distribution of any "article or thing designed or intended for . . . preventing conception," except for the regular practice of doctors or druggists,[38] the Attorney General has stated that literature pertaining to birth control is not such an "article or thing" within the meaning of the statute and thus may be circulated freely, provided it is not an actual advertisement for a trade branded article. *Op. Atty. Gen. 1970, # 70–3–35.*

Louisiana and Nebraska have statutes that refer to "secret" drugs, nostrums and medicines. Nebraska's statute prohibits sale of "secret" nostrums, drugs or medicines for preventing conception.[39] The Nebraska Supreme Court ruled in 1965 that if a nostrum, drug or medicine is not "secret," the statute is not violated.[40] Since most contraceptives are not secret, the statute would seem to have little effect upon their sale or distribution. It is interesting to note moreover that not only are contraceptives sold in Nebraska,[41] but also the State of Nebraska distributes family planning information and services to its welfare recipients, clearly indicating a state policy in favor of distribution of contraceptives, and a lack of "secrecy" with respect to those contraceptives that are distributed. The Louisiana statute prohibits the "advertising of any secret drug or nostrum exclusively for the use of females for preventing conception."[42] A Louisiana Attorney General's opinion in 1965 narrowed the effect of the Louisiana statute by ascribing to "secret" its usual meaning, thereby permitting distribution generally.[43] Before this 1965 opinion a 1934 opinion had interpreted the law as making illegal the manufacture, distribution or sale of contraceptives in Louisiana.[44]

In New Jersey, a statute prohibits any person "without just cause" from selling, advertising or displaying contraceptives.[45] The New Jersey Supreme Court has interpreted this to permit the display of contraceptives to a woman in a van parked in a municipal parking lot, incidental to an explanation of birth control.[46] Thus, display incidental to oral explanation of birth control is considered to be with "just cause."

In *Poe v. Ullman*, 367 U.S. 497, 81 S.Ct. 1752, 6 L. Ed. 2d 989 (1961), decided four years before the *Griswold* case struck down the Connecticut anti-birth control statute as unconstitutional, the Supreme Court interpreted the situation in Connecticut, where there had been only one recorded prosecution under the statute in the 75 years since its enactment and found that the lack of recorded prosecutions and the unchallenged, open, ubiquitous public sales of contraceptive devices showed a deeply embedded state policy amounting to a tacit agreement on the part of the state not to prosecute violators of the statute.

These situations typify ways in which administrative and law enforcement officials have in effect modified statutes restricting the sale, advertising and display of contraceptives despite legislative inaction.

Conclusion

Dissemination of information about contraceptives is lawful in all states under applicable judicial authority interpreting the First Amendment to the Constitution. Sale or distribution of contraceptives is permitted under the law of all states. Existing restrictive legislation, for the most part, regulates who may sell or distribute contraceptives and the conditions under which they may be advertised or displayed. The clear trend is toward elimination of state statutory restrictions.

An increasing number of states now have affirmative legislation establishing family planning programs. Some states restrict these services to the indigent; others authorize services to be provided for persons desiring them regardless of economic status.

Footnotes to "State Laws Relating to Contraception"

1. California, Delaware, Illinois, Kansas, Mississippi, Missouri, Nevada, Ohio, Washington, and Wyoming repealed their restrictive laws. Indiana, Minnesota, Maine, Massachusetts and New York liberalized their laws. Connecticut's law was overturned as the result of the *Griswold* decision.
2. Alaska, California, Colorado, Georgia, Hawaii, Illinois, Iowa, Kansas, Louisiana, Michigan, Nevada, New York, Ohio, Oklahoma, Oregon, Tennessee, West Virginia, Wyoming.
3. Alabama, Alaska, California, Colorado, Connecticut, Delaware, Florida, Georgia, Illinois, Kansas, Kentucky, Mississippi, Missouri, Nevada, New Hampshire, New Mexico, North Carolina, Ohio, Oklahoma, Rhode Island, South Carolina, Tennessee, Utah, Vermont, Virginia, Washington, West Virginia and Wyoming.
4. *Griswold v. Connecticut*, 381 U.S. 479 (1965).
5. All in *1*. above, except Indiana and Kansas whose statutes date from 1963, and, of course, Connecticut.
6. Alaska, California, Colorado, Georgia, Kansas, Nevada, Oklahoma, Oregon, Tennessee, Wyoming.
7. Illinois, Iowa, Louisiana, Michigan, New York, Ohio, West Virginia.
8. Senate Bill No. 871 Chap. No. 400, Public Acts of 1971.
9. Colo. Rev. Stat. Ann. §§ 66-32-1 to 66-32-3 (1971 Supp.).
10. Okla. Stat. tit. 63, §§ 2071 to 2074 (1967 Supp.).
11. Kan. Stat. Ann. § 23-501 (1970 Supp.).
12. Alabama, Alaska, Arizona, California, Colorado, Connecticut, Delaware, Florida, Georgia, Hawaii, Illinois, Indiana, Kansas, Kentucky, Louisiana, Michigan, Mississippi, Missouri, Nevada, New Hampshire, New Mexico, North Carolina, Ohio, Oklahoma, Pennsylvania, Rhode Island, South Carolina, Tennessee, Utah, Vermont, Virginia, Washington, West Virginia, Wyoming.
13. "Restrict" is used herein to indicate an actual prohibition, while "regulate" is used to indicate permission under certain specified conditions.
14. Note that this tabulation refers to state laws on contraceptives. Several states have separate laws on prophylactics, defined as drugs or devices to prevent venereal disease, i.e. condoms; but these are not included in these figures. Condoms can be used both for the prevention of venereal disease, and for the prevention of conception. Some question whether condoms, intended for use in the prevention of conception, would be regulated in those states with statutes on prophylactics. Most states would probably retain the distinction, with only a few blurring the distinction. See individual states profiles on this question.
14a. In *Eisenstadt v. Baird*, 40 U.S. Law Week 4303, March 21, 1972 (in which the Supreme Court struck down the Massachusetts birth control law), the question of state restrictions on distribution of contraceptives was discussed.

The majority and concurring opinions noted that the requirement in the Massachusetts statute of a doctor's prescription for all kinds of contraceptives for married persons even if the contraceptives were not potentially dangerous made the statute "overbroad." It seems reasonable to conclude that if the Massachusetts statute had not distinguished between married and unmarried persons, but had been challenged solely on the basis that it required all persons to have a doctor's prescription for all contraceptives, the same Court would have held it unconstitutional as overbroad. The opinion of the concurring Justices also suggests that a state requirement that all contraceptives be obtained either from a physician or from a licensed pharmacist would be unconstitutional. Such a decision could be of great practical importance because in rural areas, for example, pharmacies are not readily accessible. If distribution of nonprescription items such as condoms and foams, which present no apparent health hazard, were limited to physicians and pharmacists, this would effectively inhibit the ability of many persons to obtain contraceptives and thus in effect violate the constitutional right to use contraceptives, as guaranteed by *Griswold*.
15. The following 12 states have laws regulating or restricting the sale or distribution of prophylactics: California, Colorado, Hawaii, Idaho, Kentucky, Maine, Michigan, Nebraska, Pennsylvania, Utah, Virginia, Washington.
16. Maryland, North Dakota, South Dakota.
17. Hawaii and Pennsylvania have no restrictions on sale and distribution of prophylactics other than prohibiting sale by vending machine.
18. Me. Rev. Stat. Ann. tit. 22, § 2212-A (1971).
19. Arkansas, Idaho, Iowa, Massachusetts, Minnesota, Montana, Nebraska, New Jersey, New York, Oregon, Texas, Wisconsin.
20. Arkansas, Idaho, Massachusetts, Minnesota, Montana, Oregon.

21. New Jersey's statute prohibits sale and distribution of contraceptives "without just cause," N.J. Rev. Stat. § 2A: 170–76 (Supp. 1953). In several cases, New Jersey courts have assumed that this limitation applies to sale by vending machine. Iowa's statute prohibits the sale or giving away of contraceptives, Iowa Code § 725.5 (1966). An Iowa Supreme Court case held this statute applicable to sales by vending machines.
22. Mass. Gen. Laws Ann. Ch. 272, §§ 20, 21, 21A (1966 Supp.).
23. Wis. Stat. § 450.11 (4) (1969).
24. In *Griswold* v. *Connecticut*, 381 U.S. 479 (1965), the right of married persons to practice birth control was established. Since then a number of lower court cases have construed *Griswold* as having recognized the "fundamental right of a woman to choose whether or not to bear children." See, e.g., *People* v. *Belous*, 71 Cal. 2d 954, 80 Cal. Rptr. 354, 458 P. 2d 194 (1969), *cert. denied* 397 U.S. 915 (1970). A majority consisting of four justices of the United States Supreme Court held in *Eisenstadt* v. *Baird*, 40 U.S. Law Week 4303 (March 21, 1972), that "whatever the rights of the individual to access to contraceptives may be, the rights must be the same for the unmarried and the married alike."
25. Alabama, Alaska, California, Colorado, Connecticut, Delaware, Florida, Georgia, Illinois, Kansas, Kentucky, Maine, Maryland, Minnesota, Mississippi, Missouri, Nevada, New Hampshire, New Mexico, North Carolina, North Dakota, Ohio, Oklahoma, Rhode Island, South Carolina, Tennessee, Texas, Utah, Vermont, Virginia, Washington, West Virginia, Wyoming.
26. Arkansas, Arizona, Hawaii, Idaho, Indiana, Iowa, Massachusetts, Michigan, Montana, New Jersey, New York, Oregon, South Dakota, Wisconsin.
27. Eight states have laws restricting the advertising of prophylactics: California, Colorado, Hawaii, Idaho, Kentucky, Michigan, Utah, West Virginia.
28. Alabama, Alaska, Arizona, California, Colorado, Connecticut, Delaware, Florida, Georgia, Hawaii, Illinois, Indiana, Iowa, Kansas, Kentucky, Louisiana, Maine, Maryland, Michigan, Minnesota, Mississippi, Missouri, Nebraska, Nevada, New Hampshire, New Mexico, North Carolina, North Dakota, Ohio, Oklahoma, Pennsylvania, Rhode Island, South Carolina, Tennessee, Texas, Utah, Vermont, Virginia, Washington, West Virginia, Wyoming.
29. Arkansas, Idaho, Massachusetts, Montana, New Jersey, New York, Oregon, South Dakota, Wisconsin.
30. See *State* v. *Baird*, 50 N.J. 376, 235 A. 2d 673 (1967).
31. See Op. Atty. Gen. 1971, No. OP–0227.
32. In addition to those states with laws restricting display of contraceptives, seven states have laws restricting the display of prophylactics: California, Colorado, Idaho, Kentucky, Michigan, Nebraska, Utah.
33. Mass. Gen. Laws Ann. Ch. 272, §§ 20, 21 (1966 Supp.).
34. 355 Mass. 746, 247 N.E. 2d 574 (1969).
35. *Griswold* v. *Connecticut*, 381 U.S. 479 (1965); *Stanley* v. *Georgia*, 394 U.S. 557 (1969); *Red Lion Broadcasting Co.* v. *F.C.C.*, 395 U.S. 367 (1969); *N.Y. Times Co.* v. *Sullivan*, 376 U.S. 254 (1964); *Martin* v. *City of Struthers*, 319 U.S. 141 (1943); *Mandel* v. *Mitchell*, 325 F. Supp. 620 (1971).
36. One feature of a "right to hear and read" test to measure the validity of state statutes against display, advertising, and dissemination of information relative to contraceptives is that people who wish to know about contraception can initiate their own suits challenging the constitutionality of restrictive statutes; this eliminates the necessity on the part of those who wish to advertise or disseminate such information of risking criminal prosecution to test such statutes.
37. Ariz. Rev. Stat. Ann. § 13–213 (1956).
38. Iowa Code § 725.5 (1966).
39. Neb. Rev. Stat. § 28–423 (1964).
40. *State* v. *Lauritsen*, 178 Neb. 230, 132 N.W. 2d 379 (1965).
41. See T. R. Pansing, "Criminal law—Contraceptive Statutes—Prophylactic Control Act—Implied Repeal—Implied Exception," 19 Nebraska Law Bulletin 35 (1940).
42. La. Rev. Stat. § 14.88 (1950).
43. Op. Atty. Gen. 1965, p. 300.
44. Op. Atty. Gen. 1934–36, p. 73.
45. N.J. Rev. Stat. § 2A: 170–76 (Supp. 1953).
46. *State* v. *Baird*, 50 N.J. 376, 235 A. 2d 673 (1967).

APPENDIX C*

Summary and Analysis of State Laws Relating to Voluntary Sterilization

The term "voluntary sterilization" is used in this report to denote a surgical procedure which is performed by a physician upon a person who requests it in order to obtain permanent protection from conception.[1]

The most common surgical method for accomplishing voluntary sterilization of men is vasectomy, which is the surgical excision and/or ligation (tying off) of a portion of each vas deferens (the excretory ducts of the testes).

The most common surgical method for accomplishing voluntary sterilization of women is tubal sterilization, which is the surgical excision and/or ligation of portions of the oviducts, or fallopian tubes.

Vasectomy is a relatively simple procedure which can be performed in a doctor's office. Tubal sterilization via the new laparoscopic and culdoscopic techniques may also be performed as an outpatient or overnight stay procedure, but is generally performed in a hospital. The more traditional methods of female sterilization, involving the opening of the abdominal cavity, require a hospital stay of several days. (The term "salpingectomy" is generally used synonymously for tubal sterilization though it literally means the excision of the fallopian tubes). Both vasectomy and tubal sterilization are to be distinguished from castration, which is the surgical removal of the testes or ovaries, and from hysterectomy, the excision of the uterus, which procedures also result in sterilization.

Voluntary sterilization must be distinguished from "compulsory sterilization." Many states have statutes which provide for the sterilization of certain groups of people—usually inmates of state institutions who are afflicted with certain forms of insanity or mental deficiency—sometimes with, but sometimes without, the consent of the patient. These statutes are known as "compulsory sterilization laws," and are not within the scope of this study. Serious questions have been raised as to their constitutionality.

Voluntary sterilization may be performed for contraceptive (sometimes referred to as socioeconomic) reasons or for reasons of medical necessity. When performed for reasons of medical necessity, it is sometimes called "therapeutic sterilization." Therapeutic sterilization ordinarily denotes sterilization of a potential mother, on her request, because of circumstances indicating that pregnancy would endanger her physical well-being or health. Sterilization is generally regarded as therapeutic if the woman's psychological instability would seriously impair her ability to function as an adequate parent.[2]

The nature of a wife's condition may be "transferred" to the husband, as where surgery is contraindicated in the wife, or the couple decides on vasectomy of the husband as a less expensive form of voluntary sterilization.[3] It is also possible for a man to have a vasectomy for reasons beneficial to his own physical health, as in connection with prostate surgery.

In view of the broadening concept of "health" which includes mental health,[4] and the fact that voluntary sterilization for contraceptive purposes is generally beneficial to the mental health of persons who do not desire more children, the distinction between "therapeutic" and "contraceptive" voluntary sterilization would appear not to be important.

Is Voluntary Sterilization Legal?

Voluntary sterilization for all reasons is legal in all states with the possible exception of Utah and it is specifically affirmed as legal in the statutes, judicial decisions, Attorneys General's opinions and/or the state health and welfare policies of 44 states. A Utah statute may be read as prohibiting voluntary sterilization except for reasons of medical necessity.[5] A recent lower court case in Utah held that this restriction applies only to the inmates of state institutions who are subject to Utah's compulsory sterilization statute; the case is now pending for decision on an appeal to the Utah Supreme Court.[6] Similar statutes have been repealed in Connecticut and Kansas.[7]

Most states have no statute at all on the subject of voluntary sterilization. Nineteen states by statute either explicitly or implicitly authorize it. In 12 states, judicial decisions, and in eight states Attorneys General's opinions state that voluntary sterilization is consistent with public policy. Indeed, the important legal question today is not the legality of voluntary sterilization, which is generally recognized, but the right of individuals to compel physi-

---

*Source: Report of the National Center for Planning Services, Health Services and Mental Health Administration, U.S. Department of Health, Education and Welfare

cians and hospitals to perform such sterilization procedures on them.

Statutes Authorizing Voluntary Sterilization

Four states—Georgia,[8] North Carolina,[9] Virginia [10] and Oregon [11] have statutes which specifically authorize voluntary sterilization. The first three state statutes prescribe detailed procedures which must be followed. Each requires that the procedure must be performed by a duly licensed physician or surgeon who must collaborate with at least one other licensed physician. In Virginia, the surgical methods authorized are vasectomy and salpingectomy; both must be performed in a licensed hospital. In North Carolina, the surgical methods authorized are surgical interruption of the vas deferens or fallopian tubes; the surgical interruption of fallopian tubes must be performed in a licensed hospital.

North Carolina and Virginia provide that the request for sterilization must be made in writing at least 30 days prior to the operation by the person to be sterilized and, if married, by his or her spouse.

Georgia, while not requiring the operation to be performed in a hospital nor prescribing a waiting period, does have a requirement of spousal consent for married persons. All three states provide at least one exception to the spousal consent requirement. In Georgia, the spousal consent requirement is waived if the spouse cannot be found after reasonable effort. North Carolina has four exceptions. They apply where: the spouse has been declared mentally incompetent; the spouses are divorced; a separation agreement has been entered into; or the wife, who is seeking the operation, furnishes an affidavit that her husband abandoned her and failed to contribute to her support for at least the preceding six months. In Virginia, the spouse's consent is not necessary if the person seeking sterilization states in writing under oath that his or her spouse has disappeared or that they have been separated continuously for a period of more than two years prior thereto.

Each state requires that, prior to or at the time of the request for sterilization, a full and reasonable medical explanation must be given by the physician to the patient as to the meaning and consequences of the operation.

All three states exempt licensed physicians performing authorized sterilization procedures from criminal or civil liability except for negligence.

Oregon's statute specifically provides that a person may be sterilized by appropriate means upon his request and upon the advice of a licensed physician. No special requirements are set forth in the Oregon statute.

Eighteen states and the District of Columbia have authorized the establishment of publicly-sponsored family planning programs (see Summary and Analysis of State Laws Relating to Contraception). In two of these, Colorado [12] and Tennessee,[13] the family planning act specifically provides that voluntary sterilization is an accepted contraceptive procedure, and requires that it be provided to anyone 18 years of age or older who requests it (dependent on the availability of funds to implement the program). The West Virginia statute,[14] on the other hand, declares sterilization to be a nonapproved method. In the other 15 states and the District of Columbia it is not clear from the statutes whether "family planning" or "birth control services" include voluntary sterilization. (While Georgia and Oregon have special statutes authorizing voluntary sterilization, this does not necessarily mean it is included as part of the family planning program of the state.) However, the state health and/or welfare departments of 11 of these 15 states (Alaska, Georgia, Hawaii, Illinois, Iowa, Kansas, Michigan, Ohio, Oklahoma, Oregon, and Wyoming) and the District of Columbia have policies requiring or authorizing the referral for and/or purchase of voluntary sterilization for persons who wish it for purposes of family planning or birth control.

In one other of these states with affirmative family planning laws—California—is found the only judicial opinion on the question of whether family planning services include voluntary sterilization. In the leading California case of *Jessin v. County of Shasta*,[15] the trial Court construed the California Administrative Code,[16] as meaning that "voluntary nontherapeutic surgical sterilization operations, when requested, are basic and appropriate services in the field of family planning within the meaning of Section 1276 of the Administrative Code of the State of California." The trial court also held that it was "the duty of Shasta County to perform such operations when requested by persons entitled to receive the public health services of Shasta County." On appeal, the quoted language was deleted from the judgment, not because the appellate court disagreed with it, but because it was not in controversy and the court ruled that proper consideration was not given to it in the trial.

Thus, in at least 14 of the states which have laws authorizing or mandating the establishment of family planning programs (all except Louisiana, Nevada, New York and West Virginia) voluntary sterilization appears to be included among the contraceptive methods authorized in these programs; and only one of these states—West Virginia—excludes voluntary sterilization from its official family planning program.

Three states—Kansas, New Jersey and New Mexico—have statutes which, by implication, make clear that voluntary sterilization is legal in those states. The Kansas [17] and New Jersey [18] statutes provide that hospitals cannot be required to permit sterilization procedures to be performed there. (These are similar to provisions in the Colorado,[19] Georgia,[20] and Tennessee[21] statutes. Although worded differently, all five statutes are designed to ensure that hospitals and doctors will not be required to perform or permit surgery when their refusal to do so is based on religious or conscientious objection.)

New Mexico has a statute providing that if a woman has been abandoned by her spouse, the spouse's consent will not be required for "voluntary medical sterilization."[22] New Mexico also has a statute prohibiting a hospital and medical staff from setting up special qualifications for the performance of sterilization operations "which are not imposed on individuals seeking other types of operations in the hospital."[23] (Colorado has a similar statute.[24]) This type of law, while not barring a hospital or doctor from refusing to permit or perform voluntary sterilization operations, is directed against institutional barriers to voluntary sterilization such as age-parity formulas (discussed below under Judicial Decisions Authorizing Voluntary Sterilization.)

Recently enacted statutes in California[25] and Tennessee[26] provide that no contract of insurance covering sterilization procedures may be entered into which imposes any restriction of coverage based upon the insured's reason for requesting sterilization.

As stated above, many states have "compulsory sterilization laws" which provide for the sterilization of mental incompetents (and, in some cases habitual criminals and epileptics). All of these laws establish elaborate procedures which must be followed in every case. Ten of the compulsory sterilization statutes contain provisions similar to Arizona's, which reads:

> Nothing in this article shall be construed to prevent medical or surgical treatment based on sound therapeutic reasons of any person in the state by a physician or surgeon licensed by the state, which may incidentally involve nullification or destruction of reproductive functions.[27]

In other words, if an operation such as removal of a cancerous womb or prostate gland is performed on a person who is otherwise subject to the provisions of the compulsory sterilization law (i.e., a mental incompetent), the procedures prescribed in the compulsory sterilization law need not be followed although the operation may result in sterilization of the patient. By necessary implication these clauses establish the legality of voluntary sterilization performed for medical reasons on *any person*. The clauses are sometimes referred to as "savings clauses" because when there is a medical necessity for the sterilization they dispense with the procedural requirements for persons to whom the compulsory sterilization statutes would otherwise apply.

It is clear, however, that these "savings clauses" do not limit to medical necessity the permissible grounds of voluntary sterilization for persons not subject to the compulsory statutes. Thus, although such clauses are found in the compulsory sterilization laws of Georgia, North Carolina and Virginia, those states specifically authorize by statute voluntary sterilization for any reason. Other states which have substantially similar "savings clauses" are Indiana, Mississippi, Montana, New Hampshire, Oklahoma and Utah (Utah also has the statute referred to above which may be read as permitting voluntary sterilization for reasons of medical necessity only—see discussion above and footnote 5).[28]

Two states—South Carolina and West Virginia—have compulsory sterilization laws containing somewhat differently worded "savings clauses," which appear, however, to have the same legal effect as those in the ten states listed above.[29]

Arkansas' compulsory sterilization law contains a "savings clause" so worded that it clearly authorizes voluntary sterilization for *any* reason.[30]

Judicial Decisions Authorizing Voluntary Sterilization

We have found no reported case of an attempted criminal prosecution of a physician who sterilized a consenting patient.

The judicial decisions on the subject of voluntary sterilization of adults fall into two categories. First are cases in which the plaintiffs seek to compel a hospital or governmental body to perform or permit the performance of voluntary sterilization. Second are cases in which the plaintiffs seek damages for the allegedly negligent performance of voluntary sterilization procedures, resulting in unwanted pregnancies.

Suits Demanding Voluntary Sterilization

Probably the leading American case on the subject of voluntary sterilization is the California decision in *Jessin* v. *County of Shasta*.[31] The plaintiffs, husband and wife, alleged that they were unable to provide medical care and health services for themselves and were eligible to receive such services from the appropriate county public health agency. They contended that as they were already the parents of as many minor children as they could adequately care for and support, the county was required by law to furnish them with surgical sterilization. The county refused to provide the services on the stated belief that the rendering of such services would be unlawful.

The county's argument was rejected by the trial court and by an intermediate appellate court. The appellate court said:

> California has no public policy prohibiting consensual sterilization operations, and... non-therapeutic surgical sterilization operations are legal in this state where competent consent has been given.[32]

As stated above (under Statutes Authorizing Voluntary Sterilization), the appellate court did not rule on the question of whether voluntary sterilization was a health service which the county was *obligated* to provide.

Often, persons seeking voluntary sterilization cannot obtain it because of institutional barriers such as hospital rules regarding eligibility. Many hospitals have adopted an "age-parity formula" pursuant to which a woman's age multiplied by the number of children she already has must equal an arbitrarily selected number (such as 100 or 130) before she will be allowed to be sterilized. Other hospitals simply refuse to perform voluntary sterilization procedures except for reasons of 'medical necessity.' We have seen (above, under Statutes Authorizing Voluntary Sterilization) that some states, by statute, protect a hospital's or physician's right to refuse to perform sterilizations. Even in the absence of a statute, a hospital which is entirely supported by *private* funds may have a constitutional right to choose which operations to permit. Recently, however, a number of individuals have successfully challenged the right of hospitals which receive *public funds* to set up rules restricting voluntary sterilization. The ground for these challenges is that such hospitals are "affected with state action" (i.e., acting in behalf of the state) and, therefore, may not arbitrarily discriminate against a patient who seeks to be sterilized.

Thus, in *McCabe* v. *Nassau County Medical Center*,[33] Mrs. Linda McCabe sought an order compelling a public hospital and its officials to sterilize her, as well as damages for their refusal to do so. The refusal was based on an age-parity formula under which Mrs. McCabe was required by the hospital to have five children before she could be sterilized. (She was actually 25 years old and had four small children.) Mrs. McCabe alleged that she could not afford to go to a private hospital for the operation. After the suit was commenced, the hospital reversed its position and performed the sterilization. The lower court thereupon dismissed the action as "moot and academic."

The United States Court of Appeals for the Second Circuit (New York and Connecticut) reversed the lower court's dismissal of the action. The Court of Appeals held that Mrs. McCabe had stated a valid cause of action for damages.

In a similar New York suit, a hospital permitted a sterilization procedure to be performed after a lower federal court ruled that it would order the hospital to permit performance of the procedure if it failed to do so voluntarily within the time fixed by the court.[34]

The United States District Court for the District of Oregon recently handed down a decision in the case of *Chrisman* v. *Sisters of St. Joseph of Newark*.[35] Mrs. Barbara Ann Chrisman, having decided, for socioeconomic reasons, to bear no more children following the termination of her then current pregnancy, requested that the hospital allow her doctor to perform a tubal ligation during her forthcoming maternity hospitalization. The hospital refused. Mrs. Chrisman thereupon sued for damages and for an order compelling the hospital to permit the surgery. During pretrial proceedings, she obtained the desired sterilization at another hospital. The defendants moved for summary judgment, claiming among other things that the action had become moot.

The court refused to give judgment for the defendants, holding that Mrs. Chrisman still had a claim for damages and that she presented in good faith a question of substantial public interest.

The court held that the hospital, which receives substantial funds under the Hill-Burton Act, is "affected with state action, and therefore cannot engage in racial or other arbitrary forms of discrimination when deciding which patients and physicians to admit to the hospital."

The court ruled that a trial was necessary to determine whether the hospital was truthful in asserting that the refusal to allow sterilization was based on purely medical considerations. Mrs. Chrisman contended that, actually, the hospital's committee on sterilization made a value choice involving moral and religious considerations. The minutes of the committee disclosed that, in each case when sterilization operations were not recommended, the patient desired the operation for socioeconomic rather than medical reasons. The court stated that "the meaning of these social and economic considerations involves a question of fact." At the time this report was written the trial was still pending. Similar suits are pending in at least two other jurisdictions.[36]

As stated above (under Statutes Authorizing Voluntary Sterilization), two states (Colorado and New Mexico) have statutes forbidding hospitals from imposing any special requirements as a prerequisite for sterilization operations. These statutes are directed against hospital practices such as the age-parity formula plaintiffs objected to in the *McCabe* case, discussed above. They do *not* necessarily prevent the type of hospital action plaintiffs complained about in the *Chrisman* case, i.e., a refusal to perform *any* nontherapeutic sterilization. Colorado, as we have seen has another statute specifically permitting hospitals and doctors to refuse to participate in practices which violate their religious beliefs; there are similar laws in Kansas, New Jersey, Georgia and Tennessee.

Negligent Sterilization Cases

There are judicial decisions in at least 10 states in suits against doctors for allegedly negligent sterilizations resulting in unwanted pregnancies. In all the cases, the court either explicitly rejected the argument that voluntary sterilization was against the public policy of the state, or (where no one raised the question) assumed that it was legal. The issue around which most controversy has centered is not the legality of voluntary sterilization, now generally conceded, but the proper measure of damages, if any, for the birth of a healthy but unwanted child. As will be seen from the following review of the case law, judicial thought on this subject has moved from an early view that no damages could be recovered to some recent cases indicating that damages should include the cost of raising and educating the unplanned child.

The earliest and best known case is the Minnesota case of *Christensen* v. *Thornby*, decided in 1934.[37] That was a suit based on the failure of a vasectomy performed on the husband for reasons of the wife's health. The defendant doctor argued that there should be no recovery because voluntary sterilization was against public policy. The Minnesota Supreme Court rejected this argument, pointing out that, except for the few states which at that time had statutes prohibiting voluntary sterilization,[38] they had found no judicial or legislative announcement of public policy against voluntary sterilization.

The court also rejected the argument, which was sometimes raised in the early cases, that voluntary sterilization constituted "mayhem," an old common law crime which consisted of an injury making the victim "unable to fight for the King,"[39] pointing out in its opinion that voluntary sterilization "does not impair, but frequently improves the health and vigor of the patient."

However, damages to compensate for expenses arising from the birth of the child were denied in this case, on the ground that the operation was done for therapeutic purposes, i.e., to protect the mother's physical health, and not to prevent the birth of a child.

The question of damages for the birth of a healthy child following the failure of a voluntary sterilization operation came up again in *Shaheen* v. *Knight*,[40] a case decided in 1957 by a Pennsylvania lower court. Here the issue was presented squarely, because the voluntary sterilization was performed for contraceptive rather than medical reasons. The court held that the contract between the doctor and patient to sterilize the patient was not void as against public policy. Nevertheless, the plaintiff was not permitted to recover on the ground that it would be inequitable for him to have the "fun, joy and affection . . . of rearing and educating" the child while the doctor supported it.

Prior to 1967, there were judicial decisions also in New Jersey,[41] North Dakota,[42] the state of Washington,[43] Illinois,[44] and West Virginia[45] recognizing a right of recovery for negligent sterilization, but regarding as elements of damages only the pain and suffering, mental and physical, caused by the unwanted pregnancy, plus the expenses of the pregnancy and loss of the wife's services during her confinement.

In 1967, a California intermediate appellate court in the case of *Custodio* v. *Bauer*[46] went further by suggesting that the children already born might be able to recover for the loss of support and affection suffered if their mother were compelled to spread herself among a larger group as a result of negligent sterilization "should such change in family status be measurable economically."

The changed attitude adumbrated in *Custodio* was more fully developed in recent cases in Florida[47] and Delaware[48] which accepted the principle that damages may be recovered for the birth of an unplanned, healthy child. (This principle was also recently endorsed in a Michigan case brought against a pharmacist who negligently filled a prescription for birth control pills. The court held that the cost of rearing the unwanted child born as a result of the pharmacist's negligence was a proper element of damages.[49])

Attorneys General's Opinions

Attorneys General's opinions in Iowa,[50] Kentucky,[51] Michigan,[52] Mississippi,[53] Missouri,[54] New York,[55] South Carolina,[56] and Wisconsin[57] recognize the legality of voluntary sterilization for contraceptive purposes in those states.

The Missouri and Wisconsin opinions in particular discuss the applicability of "mayhem" statutes in those states and conclude that these statutes can have no possible relevance to a surgical procedure consented to voluntarily. In this respect, of course, voluntary sterilization is no different from any other surgical procedure to which the patient knowingly consents.

Minors

Generally minors do not seek voluntary sterilization, which is a permanent means of birth control, unless a pregnancy would endanger their health, or they are carriers of a heritable disease. For those who do wish it, the law is in general the same as that applicable to any other surgical procedure performed on a minor.

However, of the statutes which specifically authorize voluntary sterilization, all except the Oregon statute prescribe a minimum age. In Georgia the person must be 21 or married. In North Carolina he or she must be 18 or married unless "the juvenile court of the county where the minor resides, upon petition of the parent or parents, if living, or the guardian or next friend of the minor, shall determine that the operation is in the best interest of such minor and shall enter an order authorizing the physician or surgeon to perform such operation." In Tennessee and Colorado the individual must be 18 or married, unless (in Colorado) he or she has the consent of parent or guardian.

The Virginia statute says that the person sterilized must be 21 or older. However, the Virginia Attorney General, interpreting the new Virginia statute enabling minors to consent to "medical or health services required in case of birth control," has stated that sterilization is a means of birth control and that minors can therefore consent to be sterilized for contraceptive purposes without the consent of a parent or guardian.[58]

Although rendered moot by a new Virginia law effective July 1, 1972 (see Virginia state profile), this opinion raises the question whether voluntary sterilization is included as a means of birth control under a) statutes enabling minors to consent to birth control services; and b) statutes authorizing or approving publicly sponsored family planning programs (some of which have been interpreted by administrative departments as authorizing services to minors without parental consent).

Sometimes the statute is specific on this issue. For example, the Maryland statute enabling minors to consent to birth control services and the Georgia and Kentucky medical consent laws giving certain categories of minors the right to consent to medical services in general specifically exclude sterilization. On the other hand, both Colorado and Tennessee in their family planning acts declare sterilization to be an approved contraceptive procedure. (Both Colorado and Tennessee, however, as stated above, have statutory provisions with regard to the minimum age for sterilization).

In the absence of a relevant statute, the general rules applicable to medical and surgical treatment of minors would seem to apply to voluntary sterilization. The leading case involving consent of a minor to voluntary sterilization is the 1967 Washington case of *Smith* v. *Seibly*,[59] where the court, holding that a married minor could validly consent to a vasectomy, couched its opinion in terms of the intelligence and maturity of the minor and his ability to understand the nature and consequences of the procedure. However, since voluntary sterilization is usually an irreversible and, in the case of a woman, may be a serious surgical procedure, in the absence of a statute many courts in applying the "mature minor doctrine"[60] might be reluctant to hold that a minor could give effective consent to it, although the same court might well find that a minor could effectively consent to contraceptive services, which are of temporary effect and do not involve surgery.

Conclusion

Voluntary sterilization may be performed by a physician on the request of a competent individual in all states. In Utah, where the law could be interpreted to restrict voluntary sterilizations to those performed for reasons of medical necessity, a lower court has ruled that this restriction applies only to inmates of state institutions. (The case has been appealed.) Forty-four states, the District of Columbia and the Virgin Islands have specifically affirmed the legality of voluntary sterilization by statute, judicial decision, Attorneys General's opinion and/or policies of state health and welfare departments. Most states have no special requirements regarding procedures for voluntary sterilizations other than that they be performed by licensed physicians, and (for women) in licensed hospitals. In several states age and parity requirements for sterilization, which used to be quite common, have been prohibited by statute or judicial decision. A few states require spousal consent, a waiting period, and/or detailed explanation of the operation. Some others relieve hospitals or physicians from performing sterilization operations which violate their conscience. Increasingly, however—as reflected both in statute and judicial decisions—voluntary sterilization is coming to be regarded as a right which may not be denied, at least by hospitals or physicians which receive public funds.

Footnotes to "State Laws Relating to Sterilization"

1. The term "elective sterilization" has been suggested for voluntary sterilization which is performed for contraceptive rather than other medical reasons. See Note, *Elective Sterilization*, 113 U. Pa. L. Rev. 415 (1965).
2. American Jurisprudence Proof of Facts Ann. (1968), Vol. 21, p. 255 et seq.
3. Ibid.
4. See *United States* v. *Vuitch*, 91 S. Ct. 1294, 28 L. Ed. 2d 601 (1971).
5. Utah Code Ann. § 64-10-12 (1968).
6. *Parker, et al* v. *Rampton, et al*, Dist. Ct. Salt Lake County, Utah, Civil Judgment #195446, April 8, 1971.
7. Conn. Gen. Stat. Rev. § 53-33 (repealed effective October 1, 1971); Kan. Gen. Stat. Ann. § 76-155.
8. Ga. Code Ann. §§ 84-931 to 935 (Supp. 1970).
9. N.C. Gen. Stat. §§ 90-271 to 275 (1965 and Cum Supp. 1971).
10. Va. Code Ann. §§ 32-423, 32-425, 32-426, 32-427 (1969).
11. Ore. Rev. Stat. § 435.305 (1969).
12. Colo. Rev. Stat. § 66-32-2 (1971).
13. Senate Bill No. 871, Ch. 400, Pub. Acts of 1971.
14. W. Va. Code Ann. § 16-2 B-2 (1970 Supp.).
15. 274 Cal. App. 2d 737, 79 Cal. Reptr. 359 (Ct. App. 3d D. 1969).
16. To be distinguished from the California Welfare & Institutions Code, § 10053.2 of which establishes California's family planning program for all former, current and potential public assistance recipients of childbearing age. Section 10053.2, enacted as part of the Welfare Reform Act of 1971, is more fully discussed in the California profile under Contraception. It is not clear whether "family planning services" under § 10053.2 include voluntary sterilization.
17. House Bill No. 1307, Ch. 206 (1971).
18. N.J. Stat. Ann. § 30:11-9 (1964).
19. Colo. Rev. Stat. § 66-32-2 (1971).
20. Ga. Code Ann. § 84-935.2 (Supp. 1970).
21. Senate Bill No. 871, Ch. 400, Pub. Acts of 1971.

22. N.M. Stat. Ann. § 12-5-43 (Supp. 1970).
23. N.M. Stat. Ann. § 12-5-44 (Supp. 1970).
24. Colo. Rev. Stat. § 66-32-2 (1971).
25. Calif. Ins. Code §§ 10120, 10121, and 11512.1 (Supp. 1971); Calif. Gov't. Code § 12532.7 (Supp. 1971).
26. Senate Bill No. 871, Ch. 400, Pub. Acts of 1971.
27. Ariz. Rev. Stat. § 36-540 (1966).
28. For citations, see individual state profiles under Voluntary Sterilization.
29. These laws are quoted in the South Carolina and West Virginia state profiles.
30. Ark. Rev. Stat. Ann. § 59-501 (m) (1971) (quoted in Arkansas profile).
31. *Supra* note 15.
32. 274 Cal. App. 2d at 744, 79 Cal. Rptr. at 366.
33. Docket No. 71-1371 (U.S. Ct. Ap. 2d Cir. 1971).
34. *Caffarelli* v. *Peekskill Community Hospital*, Docket No. 71-3617 (U.S.D. Ct. S.D. N.Y. 1971).
35. Civ. No. 70-430 (U.S.D. Ct. D. Ore. 1971).
36. See Association for Voluntary Sterilization Progress Report, January 19, 1972, p. 3—"Operation Lawsuit."
37. 192 Minn. 123, 255 N.W. 620 (1934).
38. The Connecticut and Kansas statutes prohibiting voluntary sterilization have been repealed since the decision in *Christensen* v. *Thornby*. As stated above, the only state which now has a statute which may prohibit voluntary sterilization except for medical necessity is Utah.
39. See 4 Blackstone Commentaries 205-06 (7th Oxford Ed. 1775).
40. 11 D & C 2d 41 (Lycoming County Ct. 1957).

41. *West* v. *Underwood*, 132 N.J. L. 325, 40 A. 2d 610 (1945).
42. *Milde* v. *Leigh*, 75 N.D. 418, 28 N.W. 2d 530 (1947).
43. *Ball* v. *Mudge*, 64 Wash. 2d 247, 391 P. 2d 201 (1964).
44. *Doerr* v. *Villate*, 74 Ill. App. 2d 332, 220 N.E. 2d 767 (1966).
45. *Bishop* v. *Byrne*, 265 F. Supp. 460 (S.D. W.Va. 1967).
46. 251 Cal. App. 2d 303, 59 Calif. Reptr. 463 (Ct. Ap. 1st D. 1967).
47. *Jackson* v. *Anderson*, 230 So. 2d 503 (1970).
48. *Coleman* v. *Garrison*, 281 A. 2d 616 (Del. Super. Ct. 1971).
49. *Troppi* v. *Scarf*, 31 Mich. App. 240, 187 N.W. 2d 511 (1971).
50. 1932 Opin. Atty. Gen. Iowa 35.
51. Opin. Atty. Gen., Nov. 2, 1964.
52. Letter from Attorney General Frank J. Kelley to Harriet F. Pilpel, January 10, 1972.
53. Letter from Assistant Attorney General R. Hugo Newcomb, Sr. to Harriet F. Pilpel, Sept. 1, 1971.
54. Op. Atty. Gen. No. 393, Aug. 19, 1971.
55. Letter from Attorney General Louis J. Lefkowitz to Commissioner of Social Services George K. Wyman and Commissioner of Health Hollis S. Ingraham, Aug. 21, 1967.
56. 1958-59 Opin. Atty. Gen. 224, 226.
57. Letter from Attorney General Bronson C. La Follette to Thomas W. Tormey, Jr., M.D., Nov. 25, 1968.
58. See Virginia profile—Sterilization—Minors.
59. See Washington state profile under Contraception—Contraceptive Services to Minors and Sterilization—Minors.
60. For a discussion of the "mature minor doctrine," see the General Summary and Analysis of Laws Relating to Contraceptive Services to Minors.

APPENDIX D*

Summary and Analysis of State Laws Relating to Contraceptive Services to Minors

General Status of Laws Relating to Contraceptive Services to Minors

In the last few years there has been a strong trend to pass liberalizing and clarifying laws giving minors access to effective birth control services on their own consent and initiative. This parallels the general trend for laws on contraceptives (described in Laws Relating to Contraception, above) and the recent wave of laws (adopted by 47 states) permitting minors to obtain examination and treatment for venereal disease without parental consent.

No state expressly prohibits the provision of contraceptives to minors. (New York restricts pharmacists from dispensing contraceptives without a physician's prescription to persons younger than 16; but this section does not apply to doctors.) To the extent contraception for minors raises legal questions, it is primarily in the area of parental consent.

We know of no case in which either a doctor or a layman has been successfully prosecuted under any criminal statute for providing contraceptive information or services to a minor or has been held liable for damages for providing contraception to a minor without parental consent.

Under the old common law rule (i.e., the law developed in court decisions over the course of centuries, first in England and then in the United States), the consent of a parent or guardian was considered necessary before a physician could treat a minor, and physical contact by a physician with a minor without parental consent could constitute assault and battery[1] or malpractice[2] and make the physician liable for damages in a civil suit. However, these rules were always subject to a variety of exceptions, such as emergency treatment and treatment of emancipated minors.

It is a basic principle of the general common law governing the physician-patient relationship that the patient must consent to medical or surgical treatment. Certain classes of people, such as the insane, the mentally deficient and minors in general have been regarded as incompetent to give legally binding consent. With regard to the mentally retarded or insane, it is understandable why they are deemed to lack the capacity to understand what it is they are consenting to. This is true also of very young children; it is doubtful if it applies to most teenagers. As stated by Justice William O. Douglas, "[T]here is substantial agreement among child psychologists and sociologists that the moral and intellectual maturity of the fourteen-year-old approaches that of the adult."[3] The common law by and large, however, did not in early days distinguish between the infant and the mature teenager, lumping them together as "minors" and treating them, in general, as the "property" of their parents, who could make any and all decisions affecting them.

Increasingly today, the federal government and the states have recognized the rights of mature minors to make their own decisions about their lives generally, and about their medical care in particular. Thus, since passage of the Twenty-Sixth Amendment granting the vote to 18-year-olds, there has been a nationwide trend to reduce the age of majority to 18. Fourteen states have already done so. What is more, the old common law requirement of parental consent for medical treatment of minors, insofar as it applies to sex-related health services including birth control, VD treatment, and treatment for pregnancy, is being rapidly abrogated or modified both by the courts and the state legislatures, with the result that minors of any age or above a stated age often are able to consent to their own care for all or some of these services. By 1972, in at least two-thirds of the states, females who had reached the age of 18 clearly were entitled to consent to their own birth control care;[4] and about one-third of these states they could so consent at considerably lower ages, or with no age restriction at all.[5]

The courts and state legislatures have gotten away from the old common law rule through the exception for emergency medical treatment of minors, through the doctrine of the emancipated minor and by new exceptions for the mature minor and the abused and neglected minor. In addition, numerous statutes have been enacted giving broad categories of minors the right to consent to medical services in general and to contraceptive services in particular.

Emergency Treatment of Minors

Courts throughout the country have held that, when confronted with an emergency which endangers the

---

*Source: Report of the National Center for Family Planning Services Health Services and Mental Health Administration, U.S. Department of Health, Education and Welfare

life or health of a minor, a physician need not wait to obtain parental consent before commencing treatment.[6] Many courts have held that there must be immediate danger to the patient's life or health (sometimes defined to include mental health), and some have said that the burden of proving that there was an emergency is on the physician.[7]

The emergency exception, in addition to its widespread acceptance by the courts, has been codified (i.e., embodied in laws passed by the legislature) in Alabama,[8] Georgia,[9] Illinois,[10] Kentucky,[11] Maryland,[12] Massachusetts,[13] Minnesota,[14] Mississippi,[15] New York,[16] North Carolina,[17] Pennsylvania,[18] and Rhode Island,[19] all of which have statutes authorizing a physician to treat a minor without parental consent where immediate treatment is required. In addition, Arizona, Nevada and New Mexico have emergency statutes whereby persons in loco parentis may consent for minors' care in emergencies.[20]

Contraceptive consultation and service provided to sexually active minors might be construed as falling into the category of emergency treatment where failure to provide such consultation and service is likely to result in a pregnancy which could endanger the life and health of the minor and the life and health of any child who may be born. Support for this argument is to be found in the facts relating to well-known medical risks of pregnancy faced by teenage girls. These include the risk to the pregnant girl caused by greatly increased frequency of anemia, hypertension, eclampsia and maternal mortality as well as the risk of stillbirth, prematurity, perinatal and infant mortality and brain injury to the child born.[21] That child is also more likely, if it survives, to be subjected by its youthful mother to general neglect, or even physical abuse.[22] (In addition there are, of course, the obvious social consequences: illegitimacy, precipitate marriage, school-dropout, marital instability, poverty and dependency.) There is no case law on this question, since no cases appear thus far to have arisen challenging medical contraceptive treatment of minors without parental consent even though such services are in fact being rendered in many states where they have not been provided for by specific statute.

The Emancipated Minor

The legislatures of at least 21 states [23] have declared that a minor who is emancipated and/or married can effectively consent to his or her own medical care. Courts in several states where there is no specific statute have held that emancipated minors can effectively consent to their own medical treatment.[24] Since emancipation is viewed by the courts as an extinguishment of parental rights and duties, there can be little doubt that, even in the absence of a statute or judicial precedent, most courts would hold that a completely emancipated minor can consent to his or her own medical treatment.

The relationship of parent and child gives rise to certain parental rights and duties, such as the parent's right to control the child and make decisions for it as well as the parent's right to the child's earnings and the parent's obligation to support the child. The term "emancipation" is commonly used to refer to the partial or complete extinguishment of these parental rights and duties but not necessarily the removal of all the legal disabilities of childhood (such as the child's inability to enter into binding contracts or to own property or bring a lawsuit in his or her own name.[25])

> "The emancipation of a child may be complete or partial. A minor may be emancipated for some purposes and not for others and similarly a parent may be freed of some of his obligations and divested of some of his rights yet not freed and divested of others . . ." [26] "While it is often said emancipation cannot be accomplished by an act of the child alone, this is not always true. Marriage and entering into military service have been held to be acts of self-emancipation." [27]

Most often, marriage is the event that emancipates a minor. In some states, statutes provide that minority ends upon marriage,[28] but even in the absence of such statutes courts generally hold that a minor is emancipated by marriage.[29]

Since marriage is regulated by statute, the language of the statute will generally determine what constitutes a valid marriage. While the subject of marriage is outside the scope of this study, the following observations should help explain the meaning of "emancipation":

In U.S. jurisdictions, before the enactment of statutes covering the subject, the age at which a person had capacity to contract marriage was 14 years for males and 12 years for females.[30] Most states have enacted statutes substantially increasing the minimum common law age requirement.[31]

This common law (i.e., judge-made) rule was that the marriage of a person younger than age seven was absolutely void and a nullity, and that the marriage of one over the age of seven, but under the age of consent—14 for a male and 12 for a female—was "voidable," i.e., valid for all civil purposes until annulled by a judicial decree.[32] While the general view today is that marriages of persons under the statutory age of consent but over the age of seven are not void but only voidable, some statutes expressly declare some such marriages to be void.[33] However, while minors who have reached the statutory age of consent may be lawfully married, many state statutes still require them to obtain the consent of one or both parents or of their guardian before they can obtain a marriage license. Generally speaking, a marriage entered into by persons who have attained the statutory age of consent is held valid even though parental consent has not been obtained, unless a statute specifically provides to the contrary.[34]

In some states, therefore, a minor who has reached the statutory age of consent to marriage can, by marrying, emancipate himself.[35] Some courts have held that a marriage entered into against the parents' wishes will emancipate a daughter who is under the statutory age of consent, provided that she is older than 12, the common law age of consent.[36]

A minor who enlists in the armed forces of the state or nation is thereby emancipated for at least as long as his military service continues.[37] A minor will generally be deemed emancipated if he lives apart from his parents, is self-supporting and generally controls his own life.[38] A minor living apart from his parents, with their consent, may be emancipated, even though they still support him.[39] Some case law indicates that a minor who still lives in the parental home may be emancipated if he or she works and keeps all or part of his or her earnings.[40] The job must, however, be a real one; although a minor regularly employed by a parent in the parental business may be emancipated thereby,[41] the fact that he or she performs household chores or renders occasional assistance in the family business in exchange for a small allowance is not usually held to emancipate the minor.[42] A minor may be emancipated by judicial decree and some states have a special procedure whereby this can be done.[43] A minor can also be emancipated by failure of the parents to meet their legal responsibilities.[44]

Of the 21 states which provide by statute that an emancipated and/or married minor may effectively consent to medical care, at least five—Alabama, California, Colorado, Minnesota and Pennsylvania—define emancipation in the statute and, in some instances, the statutory definition appears broader than the court-made common law rule (e.g., California, Colorado and Minnesota—see "Statutes Relating to Medical Care of Minors," below).[45]

It is generally held that the burden of proving that a minor is emancipated is on the person asserting emancipation.[46] Some states, however, have statutory provisions protecting from any liability a physician or other person who in good faith relies on the representation of a minor purporting to consent to medical treatment that he is emancipated.[47]

Partial Emancipation

Whether or not a court finds that a minor is emancipated often depends on the purpose for which emancipation is asserted; courts frequently speak of "partial emancipation" or emancipation for a particular purpose. For example, courts have found minors "partially emancipated" for the purpose of keeping their own earnings,[48] of claiming Workmen's Compensation,[49] of owning cattle,[50] and in order to determine a settlement for poor-relief purposes.[51]

A New York court held that a minor who was not emancipated for the purpose of altering her property rights *was* emancipated for the purpose of consenting to medical services.[52] A sexually active minor might be held emancipated for the limited purpose of consenting to his or her own contraceptive services, although, as yet, the issue of contraceptive medical service as opposed to medical service in general has not been presented for judicial determination.

The Mature Minor

Some state courts have declared the existence of a relatively recent exception to the common law rule which has become known as the "mature minor rule." In essence, it provides that a minor effectively can consent to medical treatment for himself if he understands the nature of the treatment and it is for his benefit.[53] This rule has been incorporated in a statute in Mississippi, where the law provides that an unemancipated minor of sufficient intelligence to understand and appreciate the consequences of the proposed surgical or medical treatment may effectively consent to it.[54]

The "mature minor rule" has also been endorsed in effect by the New Hampshire legislature. A 1972 New Hampshire statute which enables minors aged 12 or older to consent to treatment for drug dependency provides:

> Nothing contained herein shall be construed to mean that any minor of sound mind is legally incapable of consenting to medical treatment provided that such minor is of sufficient maturity to understand the nature of such treatment and the consequences thereof.[55]

In a 1970 Kansas case, *Younts* v. *St. Francis Hospital & School of Nursing, Inc.*,[56] a mother sued on behalf of her 17-year-old daughter for an allegedly unauthorized surgical procedure. The daughter had been visiting her mother in the hospital when a nurse slammed a door on her finger. The resident surgeon in the emergency room operated on the girl's finger without obtaining parental consent. The Kansas Supreme Court held that no damages could be recovered. Noting that the girl was 17 years old and intelligent and capable for her age, and that the surgery was minor, the court applied the "mature minor doctrine"; it held that a minor old enough and intelligent enough to understand the nature and consequences of the proposed treatment effectively could consent to the treatment if it was for her benefit.

Similar decisions were reached by an Ohio court with respect to an 18-year-old girl who consented to plastic surgery on her nose,[57] and by a Michigan court with respect to a 17-year-old boy who consented to removal of a tumor.[58] The majority of judges in the Ohio case rejected the view that the validity of consent to medical care depends on the consenting party's capacity to contract. Instead, the judges used analogies from the fields of criminal and tort law, such as the age at which a person can be held responsible for criminal conduct and can "assume the risk" in a negligence case and the age at which a girl's consent to sexual intercourse precludes it from being considered as rape.

A 1967 Washington case, *Smith* v. *Seibly*,[59] which held that an 18-year-old married minor could consent to a vasectomy, couched its decision in terms of the intelligence and maturity of the minor and his ability to understand the doctor's explanation of the nature and consequences of the surgery.

The Neglected Minor

Almost all states now have statutes dealing with neglected and/or abused children; some of these statutes provide specifically that the court may order medical care for such minors.[60] In a number of cases, courts have stepped in to sanction medical services for neglected minors without parental consent.[61] While in earlier periods, the cases usually involved emergency treatment, such as blood transfusions, the more recent trend is to broaden the area in which the court will act. Thus, with reference to a statute giving the New York Family Court power to order medical care for a neglected child without parental consent, that court recently held that the court's power was not limited to "drastic situations" or those which constitute a "present emergency"; rather, the court will order medical or surgical treatment for a child even over parental objections, if, in the court's judgment, the health, safety or welfare of the child requires it.[62]

Statutes Giving Minors the Right to Consent to Contraceptive Services

At least nine states have enacted statutes specifically authorizing physicians to provide birth control services without parental consent either to all minors or to broad categories of minors. These include California,[63] Colorado,[64] Georgia,[65] Illinois,[66] Kentucky,[67] Maryland,[68] Oregon,[69] Tennessee,[70] and Virginia.[71] A similar rule has been adopted in the District of Columbia.[72]

The Maryland statute, enacted in 1971, gives all minors the same capacity to consent to medical treatment as adults if the minor seeks treatment or advice concerning venereal disease, pregnancy or contraception not amounting to sterilization. The Virginia statute, also enacted in 1971, provides that while 18-year-olds may consent to all medical care, minors younger than 18 years may effectively consent to medical or health services required in connection with birth control, pregnancy and family planning.

The 1972 Georgia and Kentucky statutes enable minors of any age to consent to contraceptive services and treatment for pregnancy and childbirth, but not abortion or sterilization; the Georgia provision is limited to females.

Colorado and Tennessee have both provided, as part of their comprehensive family planning acts of 1971, that birth control services "may be furnished by physicians to any minor who is pregnant, or a parent or legal guardian, or who has been referred for such services by another physician, a clergyman, a family planning clinic, a school or institution of higher learning, or any agency or instrumentality of [the] state or any subdivision thereof, or who requests and is in need of birth control procedures, supplies or information."

In 1969, Illinois adopted a statute authorizing licensed physicians to provide birth control services to minors in the general categories listed above for Colorado and Tennessee (except for minors "who request and is in need of" information or services). In addition, Illinois authorizes birth control services without parental consent for minors "as to whom the failure to provide such services would create a serious health hazard."

In Oregon, the statute states that "any physician may provide birth control information and services to any person without regard to the age of such person and a minor 15 years of age or older may give consent to medical or surgical diagnosis or treatment by a [licensed] physician . . . without the consent of a parent or guardian."

California's Welfare Reform Act of 1971 provides that family planning services shall be *offered* to all former, current or potential public assistance recipients of childbearing age (defined in the statute as age 15-44 inclusive) without regard to marital status, age or parenthood, and shall be *provided* to those former, current or potential recipients wishing such services. The statute specifically provides that the furnishing of family planning services shall not require the consent of anyone other than the person who is to receive them.

Comprehensive Family Planning Acts

As stated above, nine states and the District of Columbia have enacted laws specifically authorizing physicians to provide contraceptive services either to all minors or to broad categories of minors without parental consent.

At least nine other states (Alaska,[73] Kansas, Louisiana, Michigan, Nevada, New York, Oklahoma, West Virginia and Wyoming) have enacted laws authorizing publicly sponsored family planning programs which specifically permit, or do not expressly exclude, services to otherwise eligible minors (e.g., call for services to "any person"). In addition, Iowa and Ohio have family planning programs for welfare mothers which might reach minor unwed mothers living at home. The health or welfare departments in seven of these 11 states furnish contraceptive services to minors without requiring parental consent.[74]

Legislation Reducing the Age of Consent

The age at which a minor can consent to medical care is affected by statutes which reduce the age of majority. There is a strong nationwide trend, as shown by the adoption of the Twenty-sixth Amendment to the United States Constitution allowing 18-year-olds to vote, toward reducing the age at which a person can undertake various activities below the traditional age of 21. Of course, the age of majority has never been uniform in all states; some states, such as Arkansas,[75] Idaho,[76] Nevada,[77] Oklahoma,[78] South Dakota,[79] and Utah,[80] have differentiated between males and females, providing by statute that females attain majority at 18 and males at 21.[81]

Statutes reducing the age of majority to 18 for both sexes and for all (or virtually all) purposes have been enacted in Arizona,[82] Connecticut,[83] Kentucky,[84] Maine,[85] Michigan,[86] New Jersey,[87] New Mexico,[88] North Carolina,[89] North Dakota,[90] Tennessee,[91] Vermont,[92] West Virginia,[93] Wisconsin,[94] and Wyoming.[95] Alaska[96] and Montana[97] have lowered the age of majority to 19, and Hawaii[98] and Nebraska[99] to 20. In Delaware,[100] 19-year-olds and in Illinois[101] and Oregon[102] 18-year-olds may now enter into binding contracts. Washington has declared that all persons of 18 shall be deemed of full age for most purposes including consent to medical care.[103]

In addition, the age at which a person can effectively consent to medical care specifically has been reduced by statute to 18 in Colorado,[104] Connecticut,[105] Georgia,[106] Illinois,[107] Maryland,[108] New Jersey,[109] New York,[110] North Carolina,[111] Pennsylvania,[112] and Virginia,[113] to 15 in Oregon,[114] and (subject to certain conditions) California[115] and Colorado[116] and to 14 in Alabama.[117]

In Kansas, a 16-year-old may consent to medical care when no parent or guardian is available.[118] And in Mississippi any "mature" minor may consent to his or her own medical care (see discussion of the "Mature Minor Rule," above).

Statutes Relating to Medical Care of Minors in General

At least 11 states—Alabama,[119] California,[120] Colorado,[121] Georgia,[122] Illinois,[123] Kentucky,[124] Maryland,[125] Minnesota,[126] Mississippi,[127] North Carolina,[128] and Pennsylvania[129]—have gone beyond reducing the age of consent for medical care, and have enacted comprehensive statutes regarding the medical treatment of minors. These statutes enable minors affectively to consent to medical treatment in many situations, but the states differ in the specific situations covered.

All except California and Colorado have codified the common law exception for emergency treatment of minors, with Maryland giving a very broad definition of "emergency" (when delay in treatment would "adversely affect the life or health of the minor.")

Married minors can consent to medical care in all 11 states. With respect to minors who are emancipated, other than those who are married, the statutes vary. Mississippi and North Carolina simply provide that a minor who is emancipated may consent to medical care. In Kentucky, any emancipated minor or any minor who has contracted a lawful marriage or borne a child may consent. Other states, in effect, permit emancipated minors to consent and provide their own definition of "emancipated." In Maryland, the parent of a child may consent. In Alabama, anyone who has graduated from high school or is pregnant or has borne a child may consent. In Pennsylvania, anyone who is a high school graduate or has been pregnant may consent. California, Colorado and Minnesota authorize a minor who is "living separate and apart from his parents or legal guardian . . . and . . . managing his own financial affairs, regardless of the source of his income" to consent to medical treatment. (In California and in Colorado, however, the minor must also be 15 or older.) Minnesota, in addition, authorizes a minor who has borne a child to consent to medical services. As discussed above, Mississippi has also codified the "mature minor rule" by permitting an unemancipated minor "of sufficient intelligence to understand and appreciate the consequences of the proposed surgical or medical treatment" to consent.

In addition, all 11 states provide that minors can consent to medical treatment for venereal disease; nine of the states provide that minors can consent at any age, but in California and Illinois the minor must be 12 or older. (See discussion under Treatment of Minors for Venereal Disease, below.) Each of the comprehensive statutes, except for Colorado and North Carolina, provides that minors may consent to medical care related to pregnancy (see discussion under Treatment of Minors Related to Pregnancy, below).

As noted above, Colorado, Georgia, Illinois, Kentucky and Maryland specifically authorize minors to consent to contraceptive services; California has specifically dispensed with parental consent for contraceptive services to minors older than 15 who are former, current or potential recipients of public assistance, or who are living separate and apart from their parents and managing their own financial affairs

Treatment of Minors for Venereal Disease

At least 47 states and the District of Columbia have enacted statutes providing that minors can consent to treatment of venereal disease.[130] (The Attorney General of a forty-eighth state, South Carolina, has stated that, in his opinion, treatment of minors without parental consent is permitted under a general statute in that state providing for treatment of venereal disease.)[131]

In the preamble to the New Jersey law,[132] which was passed in 1968, the legislature stated its reasons for enacting this legislation:

> ... Since contraction of a venereal disease is subject to serious reproach within the family circle, the necessary parental consent to treatment may not be sought by the minor because of fear or embarrassment. Allowing the child to secure competent medical treatment and to consent thereto, without the necessity for either knowledge by or consent of the parent, would eliminate one of the major bars to his seeking and receiving treatment.
>
> The threat to public health from venereal disease is of such gravity that the infected person should be treated as soon as diagnosed to protect his health and prevent the spread of the disease to others. In view of the danger posed and the increasing numbers of minors infected, it is essential that this highly vulnerable segment of our population be accorded greater freedom in securing prompt medical treatment.

More than half of the statutes enabling minors to consent to treatment for venereal disease have been enacted since 1968. Similar developments in the law giving all minors the right to consent to contraceptive services seem in process, particularly in the light of the recent statutes in many states and the endorsement of this position by the American Medical Association, the American College of Obstetricians and Gynecologists, the American Academy of Pediatrics and the American Academy of Family Physicians.[133] The reasons stated by the New Jersey legislature (quoted above) would appear equally applicable to contraceptive services.

One aspect of the related public health problem caused by pregnancies among unwed teenage girls is evidenced by illegitimacy statistics in the United States for the years from 1965 to 1968. Illegitimacy rates in older age groups declined during these years coincident with the increase in family planning services available to postpartum women. However, illegitimacy rates of girls 15–19 rose by 18 percent in this period.[134]

Treatment of Minors Related to Pregnancy

At least 16 states now provide specifically that minors may consent to medical and surgical treatment related to pregnancy.[135] While this has been held by a court in at least one state to include therapeutic abortion,[136] it is not clear to what extent "treatment related to pregnancy" will be construed to include contraception, i.e., the prevention of pregnancy. The one judicial statement found on this question was that the prevention of pregnancy is not included.[137]

One Attorney General, interpreting a statute which has since been amended, stated that whether or not family planning services may be given to an unmarried minor younger than 18 without parental consent where statutory language is in terms of treatment related to pregnancy "would depend in each instance on a determination of whether the medical treatment was given in connection with pregnancy or childbirth"; he cited "the myriad types and possibilities of medical treatment which may be offered as an adjunct to family planning services."[138]

The Question of Liability for Contraceptive Services to Minors

We have seen that under the old common law rule, a doctor who treated a minor without parental consent in circumstances not adding up to one of the common law exceptions could be held liable in a civil suit for assault and battery or malpractice.[139] However, we have found no case holding a doctor liable for providing contraceptive services to a minor without parental consent and no case holding a physician liable for supplying *any* medical service to a minor without parental consent where the minor was older than 15 and the treatment was for the minor's benefit and performed with the minor's consent.[140]

Moreover, any assault thus committed was a so-called "technical assault" as distinguished from the usual assault with intent to harm. We know of no case where a physician treating a minor without parental consent has been charged with the *crime* of assault and battery. Bona fide medical treatment, even if unauthorized, cannot constitute criminal assault and battery because no unlawful intent can be shown.[141]

Many states have statutes which make it a crime to contribute to the delinquency of a minor or impair the morals of a minor or, as in New York, "endanger the welfare of a minor."[142] However, these statutes have not been applied to a physician or a health facility for providing contraceptive treatment to minors and we know of no case where a doctor has ever been convicted, or a layman's conviction has ever been finally upheld, for distribution of contraceptive information or services to minors. We know of only three instances of attempted prosecution under such laws for distribution of contraceptive information or services. In an Ohio case,[143] a mother was charged with contributing to her daughter's delinquency by advising her to use contraceptives (if, contrary to the mother's insistence, the daughter did get sexually involved). The highest court in Ohio held that the mother could not be convicted because she was exercising her right of free speech. The mother had not furnished her daughter with contraceptive devices. In the same year this case was decided, Ohio deleted the entire restriction relating to the sale and advertising of articles "for the prevention of conception" from its Criminal Code.[144]

In Virginia, a physician was arrested in October, 1971, for allegedly contributing to the delinquency of a 17-year-old girl by prescribing birth control pills without her parent's consent.[145] The charges were promptly dismissed. As we have seen, Virginia is one of the nine states which specifically allow minors to consent to birth control services. In the summer of 1971, William Baird was arrested in New York while lecturing on birth control on the charge that he was "endangering the welfare of" a 14-month-old infant whose mother had brought her to a lecture.[146] Those charges were also quickly dropped. Baird was also prosecuted under a Massachusetts law (which prohibited the distribution of contraceptives except to married persons) for giving an unmarried woman contraceptive foam at the close of his lecture on contraception to a group of students at Boston University. Baird's conviction on this charge was recently reversed by the U.S. Supreme Court on the ground that the Massachusetts statute discriminated unconstitutionally between the married and the unmarried.[147] Baird was not prosecuted by Massachusetts for contributing to the delinquency of a minor, although many of the college students present must have been minors.

Increasingly, there has been widespread federal and state recognition of the rights of minors to birth control information and services. Under the 1967 amendments to Title IV of the Social Security Act (Aid to Families with Dependent Children) and the federal regulations issued pursuant thereto, state and local welfare agencies are required to provide medical contraceptive services to eligible persons "without regard to marital status, age or parenthood." (See Federal Laws and Policy, above: Title IV A-Social Security Act, as Amended: Service Programs for Families and Children). However, the DHEW Social and Rehabilitation Service *Title IV A Services Guidelines,* issued in 1969, added the following statement: "In respect to youths, voluntary consent includes parental consent if such is required by State law."[148]

In practice, many state health and welfare departments provide family planning services to minors on their own consent. (See Summary and Analysis, State Health and Welfare Department Policies Relating to Family Planning and Voluntary Sterilization, below.) In the context of these policies, and of the lack of criminal intent referred to above, and of the many state laws which are expanding minors' rights to medical treatment, there seems little likelihood of prosecution of physicians or other authorized persons who provide minors with contraceptive information or services. For this reason, we have not discussed these juvenile delinquency or other criminal statutes in the individual state profiles.

Only one state has a specific restriction relating to the age of the purchaser to whom a pharmacist may sell contraceptives (New York),[149] and two states have age restrictions for the sale of prophylactics (Nebraska[150] and Utah[151]). The New York statute makes it a misdemeanor for any person other than a pharmacist to sell or distribute contraceptives and prohibits their sale and distribution to persons under 16. These restrictions, however, do not apply to physicians. Similarly, the Nebraska and Utah statutes prohibit the sale of prophylactics by licensed pharmacists to anyone who is not married or older than 18, except that sales may be made by physicians or upon their order.

A Note on Confidentiality

Although it is not within the scope of this study to discuss all aspects of the doctor-patient relationship, certain questions of confidentiality related to minors will be considered. A physician who provides a minor with contraceptive services must decide whether to advise the minor's parents of the services he has rendered. In many cases, the minor may be expected to object to any such disclosure.

It is a guiding principle of medical ethics that "a physician may not reveal the confidences entrusted to him in the course of medical attendance . . . unless he is required to do so by law or unless it becomes necessary in order to protect the welfare of the individual or of the community."[152]

Moreover, many states have laws providing that a physician may not disclose information derived from professional contacts with the patient without first obtaining the patient's consent.[153] In a number of cases, physicians have been held liable for damages for disclosing confidential communications acquired in a professional capacity.[154]

However, the law recognizes certain situations where the doctor may—and, indeed, sometimes is obligated to—reveal the patient's confidences. The clearest case is where the patient is found to be suffering from a serious contagious disease (mainly VD). Here the physician is generally required by state law to report that disease to the board of health, and he is permitted to disclose the disease to persons who might otherwise become infected.[155] Disclosure has been permitted in other situations as well.[156] The New Jersey Supreme Court has stated that "disclosure may, under . . . compelling circumstances, be made to a person with a legitimate interest in the patient's health,"[157] while a New York court has pointed out that the physician must weigh a "delicate balance of conflicting duties."[158]

It has been held in two cases that a physician may

reveal to the husband information obtained in the course of treating the wife.[159] It does not necessarily follow that the doctor can reveal to parents information obtained in the course of treating their child. There is virtually no case law on the question of what a physician may disclose to the parents of his minor patients; the few cases found on this subject are inconclusive.[160] In deciding this question, a court might consider the age and maturity of the child, the nature of the service rendered and the degree of risk involved to the life and/or health of the patient.

Many states have attempted to deal with this situation by enacting statutory provisions which are designed usually to protect the physician whether or not he decides to notify the parents. Confidentiality provisions are found in the different types of laws permitting minors to consent to medical care. The most common provision is found in statutes allowing minors to consent to examination and treatment for venereal disease. Confidentiality provisions are also, however, found in statutes permitting minors to consent to medical treatment for pregnancy, and in the small but significant number of statutes which apply to all medical care of minors, including contraceptive services.

At least 28 states [161] have statutory provisions regarding the confidentiality of medical treatment of minors. Before discussing these provisions in detail, we will briefly summarize them. All but four of the 28 states provide that the physician who treats a minor need not notify the parents;[162] and of those 24, all but eight specify that he may advise them of treatment given or needed.[163] Four states [164] *require* the physician to notify the parent where the minor is found to have venereal disease or to be pregnant or require hospitalization. A fifth state requires notification in cases of surgery only.[165] Two states [166] provide that the physician shall not notify the parents of any examination or test where the minor is found not to be pregnant or afflicted with venereal disease.

The six states with comprehensive statutes covering medical treatment of minors which have enacted special provisions regarding confidentiality [167] permit the physician to notify the parents but do not require him to do so. While these six statutes apply to physicians who provide minors with contraceptive services, and the statutes of three other states [168] cover contraceptive services rendered to a minor who is or professes to be married or pregnant or afflicted with VD, the great majority of states do not have statutes applicable to the confidentiality of contraceptive services to minors (since most of the statutes discussed below relate only to treatment for VD). In many states, therefore, the law provides no clear guide for the physician as to the extent to which he may or must respect the confidence of the minor for whom he provides contraceptive services.

We shall now consider in detail the statutory provisions regarding confidentiality which have been enacted in 28 states.

Six states have passed statutes regarding confidentiality which clearly apply to physicians rendering contraceptive services to minors: California, Minnesota, Mississippi, Kentucky, Maryland and Oregon. The latter three apply to contraceptive services to minors specifically. The Kentucky statute provides that a physician may prescribe for and treat any minor for contraception without the consent of or notification to the parents or guardian but may inform the parent or guardian of any treatment given or needed where, in his judgment, informing the parent or guardian would benefit the health of the minor patient.[169] Maryland and Oregon both authorize minors to consent to contraceptive services, and provide that the physician may advise the parents or guardian as to the treatment given or needed without the consent of the patient.[170]

California and Minnesota have laws authorizing a minor who is living separate and apart from his parents or guardian and who is managing his own financial affairs, regardless of the source of his income, to consent to medical care in general; in California, the minor must also be 15 years of age or older. The California statute provides that a physician may, with or without the consent of the minor patient, advise the parents or guardian of the treatment given or needed if the physician has reason to know, on the basis of information given him by the minor, the whereabouts of the parent or guardian.[171] The Minnesota statute provides that the physician may inform the parent or guardian of any treatment given or needed where, in his judgment, failure to inform the parent would seriously jeopardize the health of the minor patient.[172] This Minnesota confidentiality provision, unlike the one in California, applies also where the minor is enabled to consent because he or she is married or has borne a child or is consenting to health services for "pregnancy and conditions associated therewith, venereal disease, alcohol and other drug abuse" and where emergency treatment is given.

We have seen that Mississippi has codified the "mature minor doctrine" enabling minors to consent to medical treatment if they have "sufficient intelligence to understand and appreciate the consequences of the proposed treatment." A Mississippi statute also authorizes physicians to treat minors for venereal disease without obtaining the consent of or informing the parent or guardian. In addition, Mississippi has what appears to be a unique statute authorizing any person who has the power to consent to medical treatment for himself or another to waive the medical privilege for himself or the other person and to consent to the disclosure of medical information and the making and delivery of copies of medical or hospital records.[173] In some instances this might give a parent access to his child's medical and hospital records.

At least 18 states have statutes regarding the right of a physician to advise the parents of a minor who is suffering from venereal disease (or, in several instances, from drug addiction). Seven of these states provide that the physician may but shall not be obligated to inform the parent as to the treatment given or needed;[174] of the seven, six stipulate that such information may be given without the consent, or over the express objection, of the minor.[175]

Another eight states simply provide that a physician may treat a minor for venereal disease without the consent of or notification to the parents.[176] Iowa provides that "the physician shall notify the parents of such minor child that the child does have a venereal disease when the results of the diagnosis indicate that the child might communicate the disease to other members of his family."[177] Nebraska requires the treating physician to send a letter to the parent or guardian of any child younger than 16, and any unemancipated minor older than 16, requesting the parent or guardian to come in to discuss the child's health problem.[178] Vermont requires that the parents or guardian be notified if the child's condition requires immediate hospitalization.[179]

Hawaii and Missouri have statutes enabling minors to consent to medical treatment for pregnancy and venereal disease. The Hawaii statute requires the physician to inform the parent or guardian of any patient younger than 18 who is diagnosed as pregnant or afflicted with venereal disease; if the young patient is not diagnosed as pregnant or afflicted with venereal disease, withholding of such information must be within the physician's discretion.[180] The Missouri statute provides that the physician may, with or without the consent of the minor patient, advise the parents or guardian if he has reason to know their whereabouts. However, if the minor is found not to be pregnant or afflicted with a venereal disease, then no information with respect to any appointment, examination, test or other medical procedure shall be given to the parent, guardian, or any other person.[181]

A Delaware statute, which gives any minor who professes to be either pregnant or afflicted with a venereal disease the right to consent to any medical treatment, provides that the physician may, in his discretion, either provide or withhold from the parents or guardian of the minor such information as he "deems to be advisable under the circumstances, having primary regard for the interests of the minor." However, notice of intention to perform any operation must be given to the parents or guardian at their last-known address, if available, by telegram; but the operation may proceed forthwith if there is reason to believe that delay would endanger the life of or cause irreparable injury to the minor.[182]

Montana and New Jersey have statutes authorizing a minor who is (or, in Montana, professes to be) married, pregnant or afflicted with a venereal disease to consent to any medical or surgical care. New Jersey provides that the physician "may, but shall not be obligated to, inform" the parent or guardian of the minor as to the treatment given or needed, and may do so "even over the express refusal of the minor patient."[183] Montana has a similar provision, but stipulates, like Missouri, that if the minor is found not to be pregnant or not afflicted with venereal disease, then no information with respect to any appointment, examination or other medical procedure shall be given to the parent or guardian.[184]

Constitutional Rights of Minors

Some recent cases have developed new doctrines articulating the constitutional rights of minors. From these can be inferred the principle that a teenage girl should have the same right as her adult sister to decide whether or not she shall bear a child. The U.S. Supreme Court decision in *Griswold v. Connecticut*[185] (discussed above in the "Summary and Analysis of State Laws Relating to Contraception") has been interpreted by the California Supreme Court as recognizing a "right of privacy in matters related to marriage, sex and the family" as well as "the fundamental right of the woman to choose whether to bear children."[186] A number of lower federal courts, in holding state antiabortion statutes unconstitutional, have recognized a woman's right to determine whether or not she wishes to bear a child, at least in the early stages of pregnancy;[187] appeals to the U.S. Supreme Court have been argued in two of these cases but on June 26, 1972, the U.S. Supreme Court scheduled them for reargument in the 1972–1973 term of court. In *Eisenstadt v. Baird*[188] (discussed above and in the Summary and Analysis of State Laws Relating to Contraception), the U.S. Supreme Court struck down a state statute which, *inter alia*, prohibited distribution of contraceptives except to married persons, holding that such a limitation violated the rights of single persons under the Equal Protection Clause of the Fourteenth Amendment.

All of these pregnancy-related cases dealt with the constitutional rights of adults. There are a number of decisions by the U.S. Supreme Court and lower courts, however, in other contexts, that "children are 'persons' within the meaning of the Bill of Rights."[189] Thus, the U.S. Supreme Court has held that minors have the right to basic procedural safeguards in juvenile delinquency proceedings[190] and that public school students have the right to wear black arm bands as a peaceful protest against the Vietnam war.[191] In the arm band case, the U.S. Supreme Court said: "Students in school as well as out of school are 'persons' under our Constitution. They are possessed of fundamental rights which the State must respect, just as they themselves must respect their obligations to the State."[192]

The U.S. Supreme Court has not yet ruled on whether public school students have the right to wear their hair at any length desired; it has denied *certiorari* (a form of appeal which may be granted at the Court's discretion) in two cases where the lower courts sustained the school board's right to regulate students' hair length[193] and in one case where the lower court overruled the school board.[194]

Justice William O. Douglas dissented from the U.S. Supreme Court's most recent refusal of *certiorari* in a case where the lower court had sustained the school board, pointing out that the lower federal courts are deeply divided on this issue, with students having won in about half the cases.[195] In his dissenting opinion, Justice Douglas expressed the view that a denial of public education to a student because of his hair style raises a serious question of equal protection of the law.

In one of the cases cited by Justice Douglas, a federal court overruled a school board which suspended a 17-year-old high school student for wearing his hair long. In its opinion, the U.S. Court of Appeals for the First Circuit quoted an early Supreme Court decision as follows:

> No right is held more sacred, or is more carefully guarded, by the common law, than the right of every individual to the possession and control of his own person, free from all restraint or interference of others, unless by clear and unquestionable authority of law. As well said by Judge Cooley, 'The right to one's person may be said to be a right of complete immunity: to be let alone'.[196]

The possession and control of one's own person would seem to include a choice as to whether one wishes to bear a child or indeed obtain any needed medical service. In a recent case decided by a Utah lower court, it was held that the defendant, Planned Parenthood Association of Utah, had an affirmative duty under its contract to provide family planning assistance and services to the plaintiff and "all others similarly situated not under the age of fourteen."[197] The court held "that to deny the plaintiff and others similarly situated would be violating the Constitution of the United States."

Another constitutional argument for the teenager's right to contraceptive services can be made in a state such as California which, by statute, provides that birth control services shall be provided to all "former, current or potential" public assistance recipients (between the ages of 15 and 44) without regard to age or marital status and without parental consent.[198] Yet a bill, passed by both houses of the California legislature, which would have allowed *all* minors to receive contraceptive services without parental consent, was recently vetoed by the Governor. It seems discriminatory, and may be a denial of equal protection, for a state to eliminate the requirement of parental consent for minors from only one segment of the population, i.e., minor public assistance recipients as defined, selected on an economic basis.

Although there have as yet been no judicial determinations, other than the Utah decision discussed above, in this area, minors may have a constitutional right to request and consent to medical contraceptive services based either on a right of privacy, a right to equal protection of the laws or as part of the basic liberty guaranteed by the due process clause of the Fourteenth Amendment to the Constitution.

Conclusion

There is a strong nationwide trend toward recognition of the rights of minors to medical care. A number of state legislatures have adopted general minors' "medical consent laws" which remove ambiguous legal barriers to rendering needed medical services to minors without parental consent, barriers which often prevent minors from obtaining needed medical services.

Many states have enacted laws providing that minors may obtain medical care without parental consent in special situations where teenagers are exposed to high medical risks. Almost all the states now have such laws covering actual and suspected venereal disease, and many cover pregnancy and birth control. The trend appears to be toward general acceptance of the right of all minors to medical care without parental consent in these high risk areas. In addition, many states have lowered the age of majority either for all purposes or specifically for consent to medical care; the nation appears to be moving toward general acceptance of 18 as the age of majority, with many states setting a lower age for consent to all or some medical care.

Even where no new legislation has been enacted, the courts have expanded exceptions to the old common law rule and permit medical treatment of minors without parental consent in emergencies, where the minor is emancipated or "neglected," and, under the "mature minor rule," i.e., where the minor is old enough and intelligent enough to understand the nature and consequences of the treatment and it is for his benefit.

Although the laws of the various states and territories differ considerably, there has been a marked expansion both of the categories of minors whom a licensed physician may treat without parental consent and of the kinds of situations, notably sex-related health care, where a minor can consent to his or her own medical services.

Footnotes to "State Laws Relating to Contraceptive Services to Minors"

1. 70 C.J.S. Physicians & Surgeons § 48, p. 968 (1951); Shartel & Plant, The Law of Medical Practice 25–26 (1959); *Zoski v. Gaines,* 271 Mich. 1, 260 N.W. 99 (1935); *Rogers v. Sells,* 178 Okla. 103, 61 P. 2d 1018 (1936); *Moss v. Rishworth,* 222 S.W. 225 (Tex. Comm'n of App. 1920).
2. "While an unauthorized operation is, in contemplation of law, an assault and battery, it also amounts to malpractice, even though negligence is not charged." *Physicians' and Dentists' Business Bureau v. Dray,* 8 Wash. 2d 38, 111 P. 2d 568, 569 (1941), quoted in *Maercklein v. Smith,* 129 Col. 72, 266 P. 2d 1095 at 1098 (1954). See also *Brown v. Wood,* 202 So. 2d 125 (D. Ct. of App. 2d␣D. Fla. 1967).
3. Dissenting opinion of Justice William O. Douglas, *Wisconsin v. Yoder,* U.S. Supreme Court No. 70-110, May 15, 1972, Footnote 3, and works cited therein.
4. Alabama, Arizona, Arkansas, California, Colorado, Connecticut, Georgia, Idaho, Illinois, Kansas, Kentucky, Maine, Maryland, Michigan, Mississippi, Nevada, New Jersey, New Mexico, New York, North Carolina, North Dakota, Ohio (if mature and intelligent), Oklahoma, Oregon, Pennsylvania, South Dakota, Tennessee, Utah, Vermont, Virginia, Washington, West Virginia, Wisconsin.
5. Alabama, California, Colorado, Georgia, Illinois, Kansas, Kentucky, Maryland, Mississippi, Oregon, Tennessee, Virginia. See individual state profiles for age at which minor can consent to contraceptive services.
6. *Jackovach v. Yocom,* 212 Iowa 914, 237 N.W. 444 (1931); *Wells v. McGehee,* 39 So. 2d 196 (La. 1949); *Luka v. Lowrie,* 171 Mich. 122, 136 N.W. 1106 (1912); *Sullivan v. Montgomery,* 155 Misc. 448, 279 N.Y. Supp. 575 (1935); *Browning v. Hoffman,* 90 W. Va. 568, 111 S.E. 492 (1922).
7. See, e.g., *Rogers v. Sells,* *supra* note 1; *Moss v. Rishworth,* *supra* note 1. See, however, *United States v. Vuitch,* 402 U.S. 62 (1971), where the U.S. Supreme Court held that in a criminal abortion proceeding the prosecution must bear the burden of proving that the doctor's conduct did not fall within an exception to the rule. The opinion contains language which by implication suggests that it would be the person attacking the physician's finding of an emergency who would have the burden of proof.
8. Act. No. 2281 (1971).
9. Ga. Code Ann. § 88-2905 (1971).
10. Ill. Ann. Stat. Ch. 91, § 18.3 (Smith-Hurd 1972 Cum. Supp.)
11. Ky. Rev. Stat. § 214.185 (as amended by S.B. 309 (1972)).
12. Md. Ann. Code, art. 43, § 135 (a) (4) (1971).
13. Mass. Ann. Laws Ch. 112, § 12E (Cum. Supp. 1970).
14. S.F. No. 1496, Ch. 544, § 144.344 (1971).
15. Miss. Code Ann. § 7129-83 (Cum. Supp. 1971).
16. N.Y. Pub. Health Law § 2504 (added June 2, 1972).
17. N.C. Gen. Stat. § 90-21.1 (Cum. Supp. 1969).
18. Pa. Stat. tit. 35, § 10104 (1971 Cum. Supp.).
19. R.I. Gen. Laws Ann. § 23-51-1 (Supp. 1971) (any person 16 or over or married).
20. Ariz. Rev. Stat. § 44-133 (1967); N.M. Stat. Ann. § 12-12-4 (1967); Nev. Rev. Stat. § 129.040 (1969).
21. See R. L. Day, "Factors Influencing Offspring," *American Journal of Diseases of Children,* 113:179, 1967; Daniels, *Medical, Legal and Social Indications of Contraceptives for Teenagers,* Child Welfare Vol. L. No. 3, p. 150 et seq. (March 1971); H. Wallace, Teenage Pregnancy, *Am. J. Obst. & Gynec.,* Aug. 15, 1965; J. Grant, Biologic Outcomes of Adolescent Pregnancy; An Administrative Perspective, *Perspectives in Maternal and Child Health,* School of Hygiene and Public Health, Johns Hopkins Univ., July, 1970. See also: N. R. Butler, and D. G. Bonham, *Perinatal Mortality, Edinburgh and London,* 1963, E. & S. Livingstone, Ltd.; J. A. Heady, and J. N. Morris, *J. Obs. & Gynaec. Brit. Emp.* 66:577, 1959; J. Yerushalmy, J. M. Bierman, D. H. Kemp, A. Connor and F. E. French, *Am. J. Obst. & Gynec.* 71:80, 1956, R. Illsley, "The Social Correlates of Childbirth," paper for Perinatal Research Committee, Association for the Aid of Crippled Children, 1964; and U.S. Dept. of Health, Education and Welfare: *International Comparison of Perinatal and Infant Mortality: The United States and Six Western European Countries,* National Center of Health Statistics, 1967, Series 3, No. 6, Government Printing Office; A. Kessler, "Maternal and Infant Mortality," *Proceedings of the International Planned Parenthood Federation,* Santiago, Chile, 1967; J. Yerushalmy, C. E. Palmer, and M. Kramer: *Pub. Health Reports,* 55:1195, 1940; F. S. Jaffe and S. Polgar, "Epidemiological Indications for Fertility Control," *Journal of the Christian Medical Association of India,* September, 1967, p. 12; J. Pakter, J. H. Rosner, H. Jacobziner, and F. Greenstein, *Am. J. Pub. Health,* 51:846, 1961.
22. As to child abuse, according to one national study, 9.29 percent of abusing mothers in 1967 were younger than 20 years of age (David Gil, *Violence Against Children,* Harvard Univ. Press, Cambridge, Mass., 1970, p. 109); while only 2.4 percent of mothers 14–44 were younger than 20 (U.S. Bureau of the Census, *Current Population Reports,* Series P-20, No. 211, "Previous and Prospective Fertility: 1967," U.S. Government Printing Office, Washington, D.C., 1971, p. 29). See also: B. Simons, M.D., et al., "Child Abuse–Epidemiologic Study of Reported Cases," *N.Y. State Journal of Medicine,* Nov. 1, 1966, pp. 2783–2787.
23. Ala. Act No. 2281 (1971) (any minor who is 14 or older, or has graduated from high school, or is married, divorced or pregnant or has borne a child); Ariz. Rev. Stat. Ann. § 44-132 (1967) (emancipated and married minors); Cal. Civ. Code § 25.6 (West Supp. 1971) (married minors); 25.7 (minors on active duty in the armed services), and § 34.6 (a minor who is 15 or over and living separate and apart from his parents or legal guardian, whether with or without the consent of a parent or guardian and regardless of the duration of such separate residence, and who is managing his own financial affairs, regardless of the source of his income); Colo. Rev. Stat. Ann. § 41-2-13 (added by 1971 Session Laws, Ch. 124, S.B. No. 169) (married minors and any minor 15 or older who is living separate and apart from his parents or legal guardian and is managing his own financial affairs, regardless of the source of his income); Del. Code Ann. tit. 13, § 707 (Supp. 1970) (married minors); Ga. Code Ann. Ch. 88–29 (1971) (married minors); Ill. Ann. Stat. Ch. 91, § 18.1 (Smith-Hurd 1972 Cum. Supp.) (married minors and pregnant minors); Ind. Ann. Stat. § 35–4409 (1969) (emancipated minors and married minors living with their spouses); Ky. S.B. 309 (1972) (emancipated minor or any minor who has contracted a lawful marriage or borne a child); Md. Ann. Code, art. 43, § 135 (1971) (minor who is married or the parent of a child); Minn. S.F. No. 1496, Ch. 544, § 144.341 (1971) (any minor who is living separate and apart from his parents or legal guardian whether with or without the consent of a parent or guardian and regardless of the duration of such separate residence and who is managing his own financial affairs, regardless of the source or extent of his income) and § 144.342 (any minor who has been married or has borne a child); Miss. Code Ann. § 7129–81 (1971 Cum. Supp.) (emancipated and married minors); Mo. Rev. Stat. § 431.065 (1970 Cum. Supp.) (married minors and minor parents); Mont. Rev. Codes

115

Ann. § 69-6101 (1970) (minor who is or professes to be married or pregnant); Nev. Rev. Stat. § 129.030 (1969) (emancipated and married minors); N.J. Stat. Ann. § 9:17 A-1 (1971 Supp.) (married minors and pregnant minors); N.M. Stat. Ann. § 12-12-1 (1967) (emancipated and married minors); N.Y .Pub. Health Law § 2504 added June 2, 1972) (minor who is 18 or older or has married or is the parent of a child); N.C. Gen. Stat. § 90-21.5 (a) (1971) (minor who is 18 or older or emancipated); Pa. Stat. tit. 35, § 10101 (1971 Cum. Supp.) (any minor who is 18 or older or has graduated from high school or has married or has been pregnant); S.C. Code § 11-157 (1970 Cum. Supp.) (married minors).

24. *Smith v. Seibly*, 72 Wash. 2d 16, 431 P. 2d 719 (1967); *Bach v. Long Island Jewish Hospital*, 49 Misc. 2d 207, 267 N.Y.S. 2d 289 (Sup. Ct. Nassau Co. 1966).

25. See *Altieri v. Altieri*, 21 Conn. Super. 376, 155 A. 2d 758 (1959); *Tyler v. Gallop*, 68 Mich. 185, 35 N.W. 902 (1888); *Niesen v. Niesen*, 38 Wis. 2d 599, 157 N.W. 2d 660 (1968).

26. *Gillikin v. Burbage*, 263 N.C. 317, 139 S.E. 2d 753, 757 (1965); see 59 American Jurisprudence 2d, Parent and Child § 93 et seq. (1971).

27. *Niesen v. Niesen*, supra note 25, 157 N.W. 2d at 662.

28. See, e.g., Alaska Stat. § 25.20.020 (1962) (females only); Fla. Stat. Ann. § 743.01 (as amended 1971 Laws Ch. 71-147); Iowa Code Ann. § 599.1 (1950); Neb. Rev. Stat. § 38-101 (1969); Ore. Rev. Stat. § 109.520 (1969); Tex. Family Code § 4.03 (1971); Utah Code Ann. § 15-2-1 (1962); Wash. Rev. Code § 26.28.020 (1961) (females married to a person of full age). In California and Kansas any person 18 or older and married may enter into any contract. Cal. Civ. Code § 25 (West Supp. 1971); Kan. Stat. Ann. § 38-101 (1970 Supp.). In Idaho any male 18 or over and any female under 18 who has been married may enter into a contract. Idaho Code Ann. § 32-101 (1963). In Alabama and Louisiana a married minor of 18 or older is relieved of all the disabilities of minority. Ala. Code tit. 34, § 76 (1959); tit. 34, § 76 (1) (Cum. Supp. 1969); La. Civ. Code Art. 382 (1971 Cum. Supp).

29. *Crook v. Crook*, 80 Ariz. 275, 296 P. 2d 951 (1956); *Matter of Estate of Hardaway*, 26 Ill. App. 2d 493, 168 N.E. 2d 796 (1960); *Inhabitants of Taunton v. Inhabitants of Plymouth*, 15 Mass .203 (1818), *Rinaldi v. Rinaldi*, 94 N.J. Eq. 14, 118 Atl. 685 (1922); *Cochran v. Cochran*, 196 N.Y. 86, 89 N.E. 470 (1909); *Bach v. Long Island Jewish Hospital*, supra note 24; *In re Palumbo*, 172 Misc. 55, 14 N.Y.S. 2d 329 (Dom. Rel. Ct. 1939); *Church v. Hancock*, 261 N.C. 764, 136 S.E. 3d 81 (1964); *Smith v. Seibly*, supra note 24; *La Crosse County v. Vernon County*, 233 Wis. 664, 290 N.W. 279 (1940).

30. *Parton v. Hervey*, 67 Mass. (1 Gray) 119 (1854); *Fodor v. Kunie*, 92 N.J. Eq. 301, 112 Atl. 598 (1921); *Eliot v. Eliot*, 77 Wis. 634, 46 N.W. 806 (1890).

31. For a table showing the age requirements of every American jurisdiction as of July 1, 1965, see Am. Jur. 2d Desk Book, Document 124 (Cum. Supp. 1971).

32. An earlier view was that an infant who married under the age of consent could deny and avoid the marriage without any judicial decree. Keezer, Marriage and Divorce 204-206 (3d ed. 1946).

33. See *Duley v. Duley*, 151 A. 2d 255 (D. of Columbia Mun. App. 1959); *People ex rel. Mitts v. Ham*, 206 Ill. App. 543 (1917); *Mangrum v. Mangrum*, 310 Ky. 226, 220 S.W. 2d 406 (1949); *State in Interest of I.*, 68 N.J. Super. 598, 173 A. 2d 457 (1961); *State v. Ward*, 204 S.C. 210, 28 S.E. 2d 785 (1944); *Eliot v. Eliot*, 77 Wis. 634, 46 N.W. 806 (1890) (decided under prior statute); 52 Am. Jur. 2d, Marriage § 14 (1970).

34. *Irby v. State*, 57 Ga. App. 717, 196 S.E. 101 (1938); *Noble v. Noble*, 299 Mich. 565, 300 N.W. 885 (1941) (applying Indiana law); *Melcher v. Melcher*, 102 Neb. 790, 169 N.W. 720 (1918); *Fitzpatrick v. Fitzpatrick*, 6 Nev. 63 (1870); *Aldrich v. Bennett*, 63 N.H. 415 (1885) (under prior statute); *Berry v. Winistorfer*, 55 N.D. 310, 213 N.W. 26 1927); *Needam v. Needam*, 183 Va. 681,' 33 S.E. 2d 288 (1945). See also *Fodor v. Kunie*, supra note 30; *Cushman v. Cushman*, 80 Wash. 615, 142 Pac. 26 (1914); 52 Am. Jur. 2d, Marriage § 15 (1970).

35. E.g., *Irby v. State*, supra note 34; *Cochran v. Cochran*, 196 N.Y. 86, 89 N.E. 470 (1909); *Holman v. Holman*, 35 Tenn. App. 273, 244 S.W. 2d 618 (1951). See Annotation — Minor — Implied Emancipation, 165 A.L.R. 723, 745 (1946); Keezer, Marriage and Divorce 208—210 (3d Ed. 1946). But see *Austin v. Austin*, 167 Mich. 164, 132 N.W. 495 (1911).

36. *State ex rel. Scott v. Lowell*, 78 Minn. 166, 80 N.W. 877 (1899); *Klinebell v. Hilton*, 2 Ohio N. L. Abs. 637 (Ohio App. 1924); *People ex rel. Mitts v. Ham*, supra note 33. To same effect, for a minor son, see *Commonwealth v. Graham*, 157 Mass. 73, 31 N.E. 706 (1892). But see *Wolf v. Wolf*, 194 App. Div. 33, 185 N.Y. Supp. 37 (2d Dep't 1920) (marriage of son under statutory age of consent without father's approval did not emancipate him); *White v. Henry*, 24 Me. 531 (1845) (same).

37. *United States v. Williams*, 302 U.S. 46, rehearing denied, 302 U.S. 779 (1937); *Iroquois Iron Co. v. Industrial Commission of Illinois*, 294 Ill. 106, 128 N.E. 289 (1920); *Wallace v. Woods*, 271 N.E. 2d 487 (Ind. App. 1971); *Swenson v. Swenson*, 241 Mo. App. 21, 227 S.W. 2d 103 (1950); *Baker v. Baker*, 41 Vt. 55 (1868).

"The power of the United States may be exerted to supersede parents' control and their right to have the services of minor sons . . . [E]nlistment of a minor for military service is not voidable by him or his parents . . . It operates to emancipate minors at least to the extent that by enlistment they become bound to serve subject to rules governing enlisted men and entitled to have and freely to dispose of their pay." *United States v. Williams*, supra, 302 U.S. at 48-49.

A California statute permits minors on active duty in the armed services to consent to medical and surgical care. Cal. Civ. Code § 25.7 (West Supp. 1971). A Michigan statute which defines emancipation for all purposes provides that emancipation occurs during the period when the minor is on active duty with the armed forces of the United States. Mich. Comp. Laws Ann. § 722.4 (Cum. Supp. 1972).

38. *In re Fiihr*, 184 N.W. 2d 22 (Sup. Ct. Minn. 1971); *Brosius v. Barker*, 154 Mo. App. 657, 136 S.W. 18 (1911); *Cohen v. Delaware, L&W.RR*, 150 Misc. 450, 269 N.Y. Supp. 667 (Sup. Ct. N.Y. Co. 1934); *Harris Irby Cotton Co. v. Duncan*, 57 Okla. 761, 157 Pac. 746 (1915); *Kidd v. Joint School District No. 2*, 194 Wis. 353, 216 N.W. 499 (1927).

39. *Matter of Stillman v. School District*, 60 Misc. 2d 819, 304 N.Y.S. 2d 20 (Sup. Ct. Nassau Co. 1969), aff'd, 34 App. Div. 2d 553 (2d Dep't 1970).

40. *Martinez v. Southern Pacific Co.*, 288 P. 2d 868 (Cal. Sup. Ct. 1955); *Wood v. Wood*, 135 Conn. 280, 63 A. 2d 586 (1948); *Jackson v. Citizens Bank & Trust Co.*, 53 Fla. 265, 44 So. 516 (1907); *Owen v. Owen*, 234 So 2d 165 (Fla. D. Ct. of App. 1st D. 1970), cert. denied, 237 So. 2d 763 (Fla. Sup. Ct. 1970); *Haugh, Ketcham & Co. Iron Works v. Duncan*, 2 Ind. App. 264, 28 N.E. 334 (1891); *Penn. R. Co. v. Patesel*, 118 Ind. App. 233, 76 N.E. 2d 595 (1948); *Carricato v. Carricato*, 384 S.W. 2d 85 (Ky. 1964); *Crosby v. Crosby*, 230 App. Div. 651, 246 N.Y. Supp. 384 (3rd Dep't 1930) *Giovagnioli v. Fort Orange Construction Co.*, 148 App. Div. 489, 133 N.Y. Supp. 92 (3rd Dep't 1911); *Gillikin v. Burbage*, 263 N.C. 317, 139

S.E. 2d 753 (1965); *Townsen v. Townsen,* 101 Ohio App. 85, 137 N.E. 2d 789 (1954); *Parker v. Parker,* 230 S.C. 28, 94 S.E. 2d 12 (1956); *Foran v. Kallio,* 56 Wash. 2d 769, 355 P. 2d 544 (1960). But see *Lufkin v. Harvey,* 131 Minn. 238, 154 N.W. 1097 (1915); *Detwiler v. Detwiler,* 162 Pa. Super. 383, 57 A. 2d 426 (1948).

41. *Jackson v. Citizens Bank & Trust Co., supra* note 40; *Van Sweden v. Van Sweden,* 250 Mich. 238, 230 N.W. 191 (1930); *Williams v. Williams,* 91 N.J.S. 273, 219 A. 2d 895 (1966), *cert. denied* 222 A. 2d 22 (1966). But see *American Products Co. v. Villwock,* 7 Wash. 2d 246, 109 P. 2d 570 (1941); *Fiedler v. Potter,* 180 Tenn. 176, 172 S.W. 2d 1007 (1943).

42. *Aetna Life Ins. Co. v. Industrial Accident Commission,* 175 Cal. 91, 165 Pac. 15 (1917); *Burdick v. Nawrocki,* 21 Conn. Super. 272, 154 A. 2d 242 (1959); *Mulder v. Achterhof,* 258 Mich. 190, 242 N.W. 215 (1932); *Cafaro v. Cafaro,* 118 N.J.L. 123, 191 Atl. 472 (1937); *Estes v. Estes,* 15 N.J. Misc. 305, 191 Atl. 107 (Workmen's Compensation Board 1937).

43. See, e.g., Ark. Stat. Ann. § 34-2001 (Cum. Supp. 1969); Fla. Stat. Ann. § 62.011 (1969); V.I. Code tit. 16, §§ 231-254 (1957). It has been argued that "this is not a true emancipation," since its result is to remove the general disabilities of infancy rather than to extinguish parental rights and duties. 59 Am. Jur. 2d, Parent and Child § 93 (1971).

44. See *Robinson v. Hathaway,* 150 Ind. 679, 50 N.E. 883 (1898); *Inhabitants of Camden v. Inhabitants of Warren,* 160 Me. 158, 200 A. 2d 419 (1964); *In re Sonnenberg,* 256 Minn. 571, 99 N.W. 2d 444 (1959); *Murphy v. Murphy,* 206 Misc. 228, 133 N.Y.S. 2d 796 (Sup. Ct. 1954); *Thompson v. Chicago, M. & St. P. Ry. Co.,* 104 Fed. 845 (Cir. Ct., D. Nebraska 1900).

45. In addition to the states which define emancipation for purposes of consent to medical care: Michigan has a statute which defines emancipation for all purposes. Oklahoma has a statute which provides that the authority of a parent ceases upon the marriage of the child, and another statute which provides that a parent may relinquish to the child the right of controlling him and receiving his earnings. Nebraska has a statutory definition of emancipation for purposes of notification of parents whose child has VD (notification being required unless the child is 16 or older and emancipated). For discussion of these statutes, see individual state profiles.

46. *Perkins v. Robertson,* 295 P. 2d 972 (Cal. D. Ct. App. 1956); *Carricato v. Carricato,* 384 S.W. 2d 85 (Ky. 1964); *Cafaro v. Cafaro,* 118 N.J. Law 123, 191 Atl. 472 (1937); *Bates v. Bates,* 62 Misc. 2d 498, 310 N.Y.S. 2d 26 (Fam. Ct. 1970); *Gillikin v. Burbage,* 263 N.C. 317, 139 S.E. 2d 753 (1965); *Bagyi v. Miller,* 3 Ohio App. 2d 371, 210 N.E. 2d 887 (1965); *Detwiler v. Detwiler,* 162 Pa. Super. 383, 57 A. 2d 426 (1948).

47. See e.g., Ala. Stat. No. 2281 § 7 (1971); Colo. Rev. Stat. Ann. § 41-2-13 (added by 1971 Session Laws, Ch. 124, S.B. No. 169); Ky. Rev. Stat. § 214.185 (as revised by S.B. 209, 1972); Minn. S.F. No. 1496, Ch. 544, § 144.345 (1971); Miss. Code Ann. § 7129-82 (Cum. Supp. 1971); Pa. Stat. tit. 35, § 10105 (Cum. Supp. 1971).

48. *Bonner v. Surman,* 215 Ark. 301, 220 S.W. 2d 431 (1949); *Lottinville v. Dwyer,* 68 R.I. 263, 27 A. 2d 305 (1942); *Foran v. Kallio,* 56 Wash. 2d 769, 355 P. 2d 544 (1960).

49. *Van Sweden v. Van Sweden,* 250 Mich. 238, 230 N.W. 191 (1930); *Williams v. Williams,* 91 N.J.S. 273, 219 A. 2d 895 (1966), *cert. denied,* 222 A. 2d 22 (1966).

50. *Warren v. DeLong,* 57 Nev. 131, 59 P. 2d 1165 (1936).

51. *Inhabitants of Camden v. Inhabitants of Warren, supra* note 44; *In re Sonnenberg, supra* note 44.

52. *Bach v. Long Island Jewish Hospital, supra* note 24.

53. *Younts v. St. Francis Hospital,* 205 Kan. 292, 469 P. 2d 330 (1970); *Bakker v. Welsh,* 144 Mich. 632, 108 N.W. 94 (1906); *Bishop v. Shurly,* 237 Mich. 76, 211 N.W. 75 (1926); *Gulf & Ship Island R.R. v. Sullivan,* 155 Miss. 1, 119 So. 501 (1928); *Lacey v. Laird,* 166 Ohio St. 12, 139 N.E. 2d 25 (1956); see *Bonner v. Moran,* 126 F. 2d 121 (D.C. Cir. 1941); *Smith v. Seibly,* 72 Wash. 2d 16, 431 P. 2d 719 (1967).

54. Miss. Code Ann. § 7129-81 (1971 Cum. Supp.).

55. N.H. Rev. Stat. Ann. § 318-B:12-a (Supp. 1971).

56. *Supra* note 53.

57. *Lacey v. Laird, supra* note 53.

58. *Bakker v. Welsh, supra* note 53.

59. *Supra* note 53.

60. See Baker, *Court Ordered Non-Emergency Medical Care for Infants,* 18 Cleveland-Marshall Law Rev. 296 (1969).

60. See Baker, *Court Ordered Non-Emergency Medical Care* S.W. 2d 816 (1964); *Mannis v. State of Arkansas,* 240 Ark. 42, 398 S.W. 2d 206 (1966), *cert. denied* 384 U.S. 972; *People ex rel. Wallace v. Labrenz,* 411 Ill. 618, 104 N.E. 2d 769, *cert. denied* 344 U.S. 824 (1952); *State v. Perricone,* 37 N.J. 463, 181 A. 2d 751, *cert. denied* 371 U.S. U.S. 890 (1962); *In re Vasko,* 238 App. Div. 128, 263 N.Y. Supp. 552 (2d Dep't 1933); *In re Rotkowitz,* 175 Misc. 948, 25 N.Y.S. 2d 624 (Children's Ct. 1941); *In re Sampson,* 65 Misc. 2d 658, 317 N.Y.S. 2d 641 (Fam. Ct. 1970), aff'd, 37 App. Div. 2d 668, 323 N.Y.S. 2d 253 (3d Dep't 1971); *In re Clark,* 21 Ohio Op. 2d 86, 185 N.E. 2d 128 (Ohio Com. Pl. 1962). But see *In re Tony Tuttendario,* 21 Pa. Dist. 561 (1911); *In re Hudson,* 13 Wash. 2d 673, 126 P. 2d 765 (1942).

62. *In re Sampson, supra* note 61.

63. Cal. Welf. & Inst'ns Code § 10053.2 (1971).

64. Colo. Rev. Stat. Ann. § 91-1-38 (Added by 1971 Sessions Laws, Chapter 161, S.B. No. 230).

65. Ga. Code Ann. § 88-2904 (as amended effective July 1, 1972).

66. Ill. Ann. Stat. Ch. 91, § 18.7 (Smith-Hurd 1972 Supp.)

67. Ky. Rev. Stat. § 214.185 (as revised by S.B. 309, 1972).

68. Md. Ann. Code art. 43, § 135 (1971).

69. Ch. 381 [1971] Oregon Laws.

70. Tenn. Code Ann. § 53-4607 (Cum. Supp. 1971).

71. Va. Code Ann. § 32-137 (as amended by House Bill 378, effective July 1, 1972).

72. D. of C. Reg. No. 71-27 (1971).

73. The Alaska statute provides for information only. See Alaska profile.

74. Iowa, Michigan, Nevada, New York, Ohio, West Virginia and Wyoming.

75. Ark. Stat. Ann. § 57-103 (1948).

76. Idaho Code Ann. § 32-101 (1963).

77. Nev. Rev. Stat. § 129.010 (1969).

78. Okla. Stat. Ann. tit. 15, § 13 (1966).

79. S.D. Code § 26-1-1 (1967).

80. Utah Code Ann. § 15-2-1 (1962).

81. This distinction will be invalidated if three-fourths of the state legislatures ratify the proposed Amendment to the Constitution establishing equal rights for both sexes. House Joint Resolution 208 (passed by Congress on March 22, 1972).

82. Chapter 218, Laws 1972 (effective May 5, 1972).

83. Public Act No. 127 (signed May 9, 1972).

84. (except for sale of alcoholic beverages and care of handicapped children) Ky. Rev. Stat. § 2.015 (1968).

85. Chapter 598, H.P. 1581—L.D. 2038 (1972 First Special Session).

86. (as of January 1, 1972) Act No. 79, Public Acts of 1971.

87. Senate No. 992 (Official Copy Reprint), Ch. 81, 1972 laws (effective January 1, 1973).

88. N.M. Stat. Ann. § 13-13-1 (1971).

89. N.C. Gen. Stat. §§ 48A-1, 48A-2 (1971).

90. N.D. Cent. Code § 14-10-01 (1971).

91. Tenn. Pub. Code, Ch. 162 (1971).
92. Vt. Stat. Ann. tit. 1, § 173 (as amended by Act No. 90, Public Acts of 1971).
93. Chapter 61, Acts of the Legislature, Regular Session, 1972.
94. Wis. Laws 1971, ch. 213 (effective March 23, 1972).
95. Wyo. Stat. Ann. § 14-1.1 (Cum. Supp. 1971) (contingent on November, 1972 referendum).
96. (any person at 19 and any female at marriage) Alaska Stat. §§ 25.20.010, 25.20.020 (1962).
97. Mont. Rev. Codes § 64-101 (Cum. Supp. 1971).
98. Hawaii Rev. Laws § 577.1 (1968).
99. (minority ends at age 20, or earlier upon marriage) Neb. Rev. Stat. § 38-101 (1969).
100. Del. Code Ann. tit. 6, § 2705 (1969).
101. Public Act 77-1229 (approved August 24, 1971). This act reduces the age of majority for some purposes to 18, including the age at which minors can enter into valid contracts (but not marriage contracts).
102. Ch. 726 [1971] Oregon Laws 1624.
103. Wash. Rev. Code § 26.28.010 (1971 Cum. Supp.); also see Wash. Laws, 1971, 1st Ex. Sess. Ch. 292, § 2 (5).
104. Colo. Rev. Stat. Ann. § 41-2-13 (added by 1971 Session Laws, Chapter 124, S.B. No. 169).
105. Pub. Act 304 (effective Oct. 1, 1971).
106. Ga. Code Ann. § 88-2904 (1971).
107. Ill. Ann. Stat. Ch. 91, § 18.1 (Smith-Hurd 1972 Cum. Supp.).
108. Md. Ann. Code art. 43, § 135 (1971).
109. See note 87 supra.
110. N.Y. Pub. Health Law § 2504 (signed by Governor Rockefeller June 2, 1972).
111. N.C. Gen. Stat. § 90-21.5 (1971).
112. Pa. Stat. tit. 35, § 10101 (1969).
113. House Bill 378, effective July 1, 1972.
114. Ch. 381 [1971] Oregon Laws 551.
115. The minor must live separate and apart from his parents and manage his own financial affairs, regardless of the source of his income. Cal. Civ. Code § 34.6 (West Supp. 1971).
116. Colo. Rev. Stat. Ann. § 41-2-13 (added by 1971 Session Laws, Chapter 124, S.B. No. 169).
117. Act No. 2281 (1971).
118. Kan. Stat. Ann. § 38-123b (1970 Supp.).
119. Act No. 2281 (1971).
120. Cal. Civ. Code §§ 25.6, 25.7, 34.5, 34.6, 34.7 (West Supp. 1971).
121. Colo. Rev. Stat. Ann. § 41-2-13 (added by 1971 Session Laws, Chapter 124, S.B. No. 169).
122. Ga. Code Ann. Ch. 88-29 (1971).
123. Ill. Ann. Stat. Ch. 91, §§ 18.1-18.7 (Smith-Hurd 1966 and Supp. 1972).
124. Ky. Rev. Stat. § 214.185 (as revised by S.B. 309, 1972).
125. Md. Ann. Code art. 43, § 135 (1971).
126. S.F. No. 1496, Ch. 544 (1971).
127. Miss. Code Ann. § 7129-81 et seq. (1971 Cum. Supp.).
128. N.C. Gen. Stat. §§ 90-21.1—90-21.5 (as amended 1971).
129. Pa. Stat. tit. 35, §§ 10101-10105 (1969).
130. All except South Carolina, Wisconsin and Wyoming. For citations, see individual state profiles.
131. 1959-60 Opinions of Attorney General of South Carolina 231 (Opin. No. 685, Aug. 5, 1960). A similar opinion has been expressed by the Attorney General of the Virgin Islands. See Virgin Islands profile.
132. N.J. Stat. Ann. § 9:17 A-4 (1971 Cum. Supp.).
133. See discussion in H. F. Pilpel and N. F. Wechsler, "Birth Control, Teen-Agers and the Law: A New Look, 1971," Family Planning Perspectives, Vol. 3, No. 3, July 1971, p. 43.
134. P. Cutright, Testimony before the Commission on Population Growth and the American Future, May 27, 1971.

135. Alabama, Alaska (examination only), California, Delaware, Georgia, Hawaii, Kansas, Kentucky, Maryland, Minnesota, Missippi, Missouri, New Jersey, New Mexico (examination and diagnosis), Pennsylvania and Virginia. The District of Columbia also has such a provision. In addition, Alabama, Illinois, Montana and New Jersey laws provide that pregnant minors may consent to all medical and surgical care. For citations, see the individual state profiles below.
136. Ballard v. Anderson, 4 Cal. 3d 873, 484 P. 2d 1345 (1971). Three of the statutes providing for medical care of minors related to pregnancy—Georgia's, Kentucky's and Missouri's—specifically exclude abortion. The Delaware statute, on the other hand, specifically authorizes "lawful therapeutic procedures [which] include abortion as permitted under the law of this State and any subsequent amendments thereof."
137. Ballard v. Anderson, supra note 136.
138. Letter from Attorney General Arthur K. Bolton to Dr. John H. Venable, Director, Georgia Dep't of Public Health, Nov. 3, 1971. In Georgia, however, a new statute authorizes services to minors for the prevention of pregnancy without parental consent. See Georgia profile.
139. See footnotes 1 and 2 supra.
140. There have been cases where physicians have been found liable for damages for providing medical treatment to a minor younger than 15 (e.g., Zoski v. Gaines, supra note 1, where the minor was nine years old), or where the treatment was not for the benefit of the minor (e.g., Zaman v. Schultz, 19 Pa. D. & C. 309 (1933), involving the donating of blood, and Bonner v. Moran, supra note 53, involving the donation of a skin graft).
141. Mohr v. Williams, 95 Minn. 261, 104 N.W. 12 (1905), overruled on other grounds, Benzel v. Halvorson, 248 Minn. 527, 80 N.W. 2d 854 (1957).
142. See, e.g., Cal. Penal Code § 272 (West 1970); Neb. Rev. Stat. § 28-477 (1956); N.Y. Penal Code § 260.10 (McKinney Cum. Supp. 1971).
143. Ohio v. McLaughlin, 4 Ohio App. 2d 327, 212 N.E. 2d 635 (1965).
144. See Ohio profile—Contraception—2. Laws and Court Decisions Relating to Sale and Distribution of Contraceptives.
145. Richmond Times-Dispatch, October 30, 1971.
146. New York Post, August 7, 1971, p. 3.
147. Eisenstadt v. Baird, 40 U.S. Law Week 4303 (March 21, 1972). See discussion in Summary and Analysis of State Laws Relating to Contraception and Massachusetts profile.
148. § 220.21. Family Planning Services.
149. N.Y. Educ. Law § 6811 (McKinney Supp. 1971).
150. Neb. Stat. § 71-1112 (1967).
151. Utah Code Ann. § 58-19-9 (1953).
152. Principles of Medical Ethics of the American Medical Association, Section 9 (1971).
153. See 8 Wigmore, Evidence § 2380 (McNaughton rev. 1961); DeWitt, Privileged Communications Between Physician and Patient, 447 et seq. (1958); Shartel & Plant, The Law of Medical Practice 48-49 (1959); Note, "Legal Protection of the Confidential Nature of the Physician-Patient Relationship," 52 Col. L. Rev. 383 (1952). Many but not all of these laws preclude only disclosures made on a witness stand. Other statutes provide that "betrayal of professional secrets" shall be a ground for revoking a physician's license.
154. See Munzer v. Blaisdell, 183 Misc. 773, 49 N.Y.S. 2d 915 (Sup. Ct. N.Y. Co. 1944), aff'd without opinion, 269 App. Div. 970, 58 N.Y.S. 2d 359 (1st Dep't 1945); Griffin v. Medical Society of State of N.Y., 7 Misc. 549, 11 N.Y.S. 2d 109 (Sup. Ct. N.Y. Co. 1939); Alpin v. Morton, 21

Ohio St. 536 (Ohio Sup. Ct. 1871); *Hammonds v. Aetna Casualty & Surety Co.*, 237 F. Supp. 96 (N.D. Ohio 1965), motions overruled, 243 F. Supp. 793 (N.D. Ohio 1965); *Smith v. Driscoll*, 94 Wash. 441, 162 Pac. 572 (1917). But see *Quarles v. Sutherland*, 215 Tenn. 651, 389 S.W. 2d 249 (1965).
155. *Simonsen v. Swenson*, 104 Neb. 224, 177 N.W. 831 (1920).
156. *Hague v. Williams*, 37 N.J. 328, 181 A. 2d 345 (1962); *Clark v. Geraci*, 29 Misc. 2d 791, 208 N.Y.S. 2d 564 (Sup. Ct. Kings Co. 1960); *Berry v. Moench*, 8 Utah 2d 191, 331 P. 2d 814 (1958).
157. *Hague v. Williams, supra* note 156, 181 A. 2d at 349.
158. *Clark v. Geraci, supra* note 156, 208 N.Y.S. 2d at 567.
159. *Pennison v. Provident Life & Accident Ins. Co.*, 154 So. 2d 617 (La. App. 1963), writ refused 244 La. 1019, 156 So. 2d 226 (1963); *Curry v. Corn*, 52 Misc. 2d 1035, 277 N.Y.S. 2d 470 (Sup. Ct. Nassau Co. 1966).
160. In *Alpin v. Morton*, 21 Ohio St. 536 (Ohio Sup. Ct. 1871), a physician was held liable for slander for having told the mother of an unmarried 16-year-old girl and two other ladies that the girl was pregnant "and that if she was not that she had got rid of it." While the action was pending, the girl died, and damages were ultimately recovered by the mother on behalf of the estate. In *Kenny v. Gurley*, 208 Ala. 623, 95 So. 34 (1923), it was held that a physician who was the medical director of a college had a conditional privilege to advise the parents of a student who was expelled that she had a venereal disease. The lower court had awarded the girl damages for libel, but the Alabama Supreme Court reversed, holding that she could recover only by proving malice on the doctor's part.
161. Arkansas, California, Colorado, Delaware, Florida, Georgia, Hawaii, Illinois, Iowa, Kansas, Kentucky, Louisiana, Maine, Maryland, Michigan, Minnesota, Mississippi, Missouri, Montana, New Hampshire, New Jersey, New York, Oregon, South Dakota, Tennessee, Vermont and West Virginia. See citations below.
162. All but Hawaii, Iowa, Nebraska and Vermont.
163. Arkansas, Caliornia, Colorado, Delaware, Florida, Georgia, Illinois, Kansas, Kentucky, Louisiana, Maryland, Michigan, Minnesota, Missouri, Montana, New Jersey and Oregon.
164. Hawaii, Iowa, Nebraska and Vermont.
165. Delaware.
166. Montana and Missouri.
167. Caliornia, Kentucky, Maryland, Minnesota, Mississippi and Oregon.
168. Delaware, Montana and New Jersey.
169. Ky. Rev. Stat. § 214.185 (as amended by S.B. 309 (1972)).
170. Md. Ann. Code art. 43, § 135 (1971); Ch. 381 [1971] Oregon Laws 551. The Maryland law specifies that the doctor shall not be obligated to inform the parent.
171. Cal. Civ. Code § 34.6 (West Supp. 1971).
172. S.F. No. 1496, Ch. 544 § 144.346 (1971).
173. Miss. Code Ann. § 7129-85 (Cum. Supp. 1971).
174. Ark. Stat. Ann. § 82-631 (Cum. Supp. 1971); Fla. Stat. Ann. § 384.061 (as amended effective Oct. 1, 1971); Ga. Code Ann. § 74-104.3 (Cum. Supp. 1971); Ill. Ann. Stat. ch. 91, § 18.5 (Smith-Hurd Cum. Supp. 1972); Kan. Stat. Ann. § 65-2892 (Supp. 1970); La. Rev. Stat. § 40:1065.1 (Cum. Supp. 1971); Mich. Comp. Laws Ann. § 329.221 (Cum. Supp. 1972).
175. All except Illinois. The Florida statute requires the physician to "make a sincere attempt to persuade the minor to permit him to divulge the nature of the condition to the parent or parents of the minor." However, if the attempt fails the physician is empowered to tell the parents anyway.
176. Colo. Rev. Stat. Ann. § 66-9-2 (4) (Supp. 1967); Maine Rev. Stat. Ann. tit. 32, § 3154 (Cum. Supp. 1972); Miss. Code Ann. § 8893.7 (Cum. Supp. 1971); N.H. Rev. Stat. Ann. § 141:11-a (added by laws of 1972, ch. 11); N.Y. Pub. Health Law § 2305 (McKinney 1971); S. Dak. Comp. Laws § 34-223-17 (Supp. 1971) (limited to doctors attached to state and county health departments); Tenn. Code Ann. § 53-1104 (Cum. Supp. 1971); W. Va. Code Ann. § 16-4-10 (Cum. Supp. 1972).
177. Iowa Code Ann. § 140.9 (1972). But a doctor may not disclose to a parent the fact that his child is being treated for drug addiction. Iowa Code Ann. § 224 A.2 (Cum. Supp. 1972).
178. Neb. Rev. Stat. § 1120 (1967).
179. Vt. Stat. Ann. tit. 18, § 4226 (Cum. Supp. 1971).
180. Hawaii Rev. Laws § 577A-3 (Supp. 1971).
181. Mo. Rev. Stat. § 431.062 (1971 Supp.).
182. Del. Code Ann. tit. 13, § 708 (Cum. Supp. 1970).
183. N.J. Stat. Ann. § 9:17A-5 (Supp. 1971).
184. Mont. Rev. Codes § 69-6102 (1970).
185. 381 U.S. 479 (1965).
186. *People v. Belous*, 71 Cal. 2d 954, 80 Cal. Reptr. 354, 458 P. 2d 194 (Sup. Ct. Cal. 1969), cert. denied 397 U.S. 915 (1970).
187. *Doe v. Scott*, 321 F. Supp, 1385 (N.D. Ill. 1971); *Roe v. Wade*, 314 F. Supp. 1217 (N.D. Tex. 1970).
188. 40 U.S. Law Week 4303 (March 21, 1972).
189. See dissenting opinion of Justice William O. Douglas in *Wisconsin v. Yoder*, U.S. Supreme Court No. 70-110, May 15, 1972.
190. In re *Gault*, 387 U.S. 1 (1967); In re *Winship*, 397 U.S. 358 (1970).
191. *Tinker v. Des Moines Community School*, 393 U.S. 503 (1969).
192. *Id.* at 511.
193. *Olff v. East Side Union High School District*, 445 F. 2d 932 (9th Cir. 1971), cert. denied 40 U.S. Law Week 3332 (1/18/72); *Jackson v. Dorrier*, 424 F. 2d 213 (6th Circ. 1970), cert. denied, 400 U.S. 850 (1970).
194. *Breen v. Kahl*, 419 F. 2d 1034 (7th Cir. 1969), cert. denied, 398 U.S. 937 (1970).
195. See cases cited in footnote 5 to Justice Douglas's dissenting opinion in *Olff v. East Side Union High School District*, 40 U.S. Law Week 3332 (1/18/72) and in *Note*, 84 Harv. L. Rev. 1702, 1703 n. 4 (1971). See also Justice Douglas's dissenting opinion in *Wisconsin v. Yoder, supra* note 189.
196. *Richards v. Thurston*, 424 F. 2d 1281 at 1285 (1st Cir. 1970), quoting from *Union Pacific Ry. v. Botsford*, 141 U.S. 250, 251 (1891).
197. *Jane Doe et al v. Planned Parenthood Association of Utah*, District Court of Salt Lake County No. 204803, Memorandum Decision by Judge Hanson, May 15, 1972.
198. Cal. Welf. & Inst'ns. Code § 10053.2 (1971).

INDEX

Abortion
    cases, 20-25
    common law, 2
    constitutionality, 20-22
    definition, 1
    reform, 17
    state laws, 2-5, 7, 10, 12
    (see also, Appendix A, Model State Penal Code)

Artificial insemination
    cases, 70-71
    future of, 72
    legality, 69
    state laws, 73-75

Comstock Act
    in general, 29
    judicial construction, 32
    cases, 32-34

Contraceptive materials
    constitutional challenges, 64-65
    federal laws, 34
    regulatory legislation, 45; 53-54 (advertising), 55-60 (vending machines sales)
    State laws, see Appendix B

Sterilization
    common law, 79
    compulsory, 79
    definitions, 77
    procedures, 77-78
    state laws, see Appendix C

Vasectomy, 78